I0429525

FROM MADHOUSE
TO MENTAL HEALTH

By

Harvey J. Widroe, M.D.

With Ron Kenner

CreateSpace 2011

ISBN: 1461112079
ISBN-13: 9781461112075

To Melanie

CONTENTS

I. RECORDING A BURIED HISTORY

It was my good luck to have been there—on the spot in 1959, the year that the slow drip of impending change in psychiatric treatment became a tumultuous torrent. At the time it felt as though a dam had burst, with the inevitable inundation of a whole field of barely effective, totally ineffective, or sometimes even dangerous therapeutics. The old treatments, ranging from psychoanalysis to insulin coma to lobotomy were replaced in short order by a new dimension of far more successful and humane psychiatric treatment—psychiatric drugs combined with a variety of supportive psychotherapies.

Before that we had endured the era of the madhouse, itself an improvement over the centuries of a lifetime in chains, or the burning of the mentally ill as witches. Each had been society's final solution to the ever-present question of what to do with seriously ill psychiatric patients.

It seemed so odd to me that even now, in the twenty-first century, the brutal and inhumane answer to the problem of mental illness apparently was still with us. "Look out there, folks! To your right is St Thomas Hospital for the Insane. Watch out if you see someone strange climbing over the wall and coming toward the bus." Some of the passengers on our double decker tour bus laughed lamely at the driver's feeble attempt at humor. Having just stopped to sample the liquid pleasures of one of Europe's larger breweries, they needed little prompting to elicit grossly inappropriate laughter. The brewery, not the psychiatric hospital, was starred on the map as one of the highlights of our tour.

The mental hospital, a relic from another time, wasn't even on the map. The tour bus driver slowed for a quick look, but offered no further comment. I was relieved that he had made no serious effort to stop. We drove past a somber greystone medieval fortress-like structure set far back behind an eight foot concrete wall that enclosed several acres. Thank goodness I didn't see anyone at all. I hoped it had been closed down the way Manteno State Hospital and scores of other institutions for the insane had been closed down. It was Manteno where some decades earlier, as a medical student, I had spent three life-changing months. Evidently St Thomas Hospital was only a minor tourist attraction. It wasn't really like a trip to Bedlam in the nineteenth century when an amusing day out to visit the lunatic asylum had indeed once ranked high as an entertainment venue. That kind of 'fun' had disappeared long ago.

Yet I was upset that the psychiatric hospital was mentioned in such a disparaging way in the tour guide's patter. I was irritated that what was or might have been a home of human suffering was being mocked, its pathetic existence still regarded as a form of amusement. In my mind I could look beyond the walls to see the inmates who had once been there; malnourished creatures chained to the walls, naked or in rags, screaming and being beaten by sadistic keepers.

When I calmed down, I could see that pleasure tours of the 'nut house' itself were truly part of the past, that what I was observing on the bus tour was just a vestige of a hideous bygone era. The laughter on our tour bus had been only a thinly disguised expression of fear of the mentally ill, tempered by the comforting belief that the lunatics were all safely locked up. The laughter was to assure us that we were safe from the crazies who even now might be lurking behind the fortress walls.

Philippe Pinel was supposed to have fixed all that awful stuff in France in the early 1800s by removing the chains from the mentally ill and then substituting more humane strait jackets instead. He and his associate, Pussin, were supposed to have done away with all of the torture and a lot more. They did get rid of the bleeding, purging and blistering—all presumed treatments for the excoriation of demons or the elimination of toxic phlegm. Treatment was to have become more kindly, with rest and talking as the major modes of treatment.

Shortly thereafter in the United States Dorthea Dix campaigned successfully for the establishment of state mental hospitals. And, starting with the New Jersey State Lunatic Asylum in 1848, she was more successful than she had ever dreamed. State mental hospitals became commonplace as the repository for the mentally ill. Their popularity as the solution to a difficult societal problem grew and grew. The populations of these facilities multiplied to unheard of and totally unintended levels. Imagine 9000 patients in a single hospital! And then multiply that number of hospitals by nearly one hundred with at least one almost that size in every state.

Not that long ago, as recently as the 1950s, jam–packed madhouses in the United States did exist. Although known then by the more benign name of state mental hospitals, they had degenerated once again to become truly hospitals of horror.

In 1956 the state mental hospitals in the United States housed more than 800,000 admitted, more often committed, and mostly imprisoned severely-ill psychiatric patients. The vast majority of the patients had little hope of ever gaining freedom from the madhouses that barely maintained them. And they had even less hope of freedom from the nonstop nightmares of the mental illnesses from which they could not awaken.

The state mental hospitals were located all over the place, but usually out of town, or on the fringe of a town whose only excuse to exist was to provide housing for some of the hospital employees. Like the inhabitants of the towns surrounding the World War II concentration camps where extermination was a daily business, those people who lived near the state mental hospitals claimed they didn't really know what was going on there. And they usually didn't care, except that the existence of the state hospital meant full employment for the townsfolk. The state hospitals, a poorly paying, labor intensive industry, were apparently immune to the economic vicissitudes that seemed to periodically affect the rest of the country. When the coal mines closed in southern Illinois and Kentucky, the state mental hospitals further north provided a work opportunity for those whose lack of skill made them unsuitable for work elsewhere.

What the townsfolk and the rest of us didn't want to know or care about was what was happening to these three quarters of a million patients. Once they arrived at the hospitals they were no longer regarded as people, but more like livestock of some nonhuman species. It is true that, unlike the concentration camps, they were not branded or tattooed. Yet, like cattle, they were largely penned into very crowded quarters. The designers of the state hospitals had not foreseen that their populations would grow to greatly exceed their intended capacities. A hospital built to house up to 6,000 patients could almost as easily hold 8,000 or 9,000 patients. Their occupants were ware-housed at best, commonly mistreated, and sometimes even tortured at worst, albeit for the most part with little conscious malice by their keepers, those who, like concentration camp guards, were just doing their jobs. And who was going to complain about it?

In 1956 I was a junior medical student, very interested in psychiatry and seeking experience I could never obtain merely by reading psychiatric textbooks. It was then that I came to live at Manteno State Hospital, in Manteno Illinois, one of the largest mental hospitals in the United States. More than 8000 mentally ill patients were kept there, most of them never to emerge.

It was all too easy for a troubled person to get into Manteno. Where else was our society to put the mentally ill who had been picked up by the Chicago police for violent, self destructive or bizarre and annoying behavior? The commitment process was quick and efficient. No patient's rights advocates argued for patients to be released. Once the commitment process was over, usually a matter of a few minutes, it was off to the blue bus that provided transport to Manteno. How else to keep the streets free of the sight of the chronically psychotic mentally ill and their potential danger to the rest of us?

II. LIFE AND DEATH IN THE MADHOUSE

They seemed dead, all sixteen of them, men and women strapped into tubs in a colorless misty cold storage room. Only their heads were visible, sticking up through an opening in the canvas cloth tightly pulled over the top of each tub. Whatever noises they made, cries, groans, and curses, were drowned out by the much louder nonstop sounds of bubbling water. The room itself, a large gray cavern, was barely lit by a few rays of daylight filtering in from a single window near the ceiling.

An attendant wearing a gray rubber apron explained that this was the hydrotherapy room. Patients who had become violent elsewhere in the hospital were transferred here from other units. "They comes in crazy and all trussed up." They would usually spend about a week or two in cold water tubs until they settled down, the attendant explained nonchalantly.

My presence in the hydrotherapy room was part of an almost self-guided tour of parts of the hospital, following a list provided by Dr Chermack, the superintendent of Manteno. My mind had been stunned by what I was seeing that morning, and my capacity for objective critical appraisal of anything whatsoever had been overwhelmed much earlier by intense waves of disgust, revulsion, and outright horror. The questions I should have asked there, and in many of the other units I visited, didn't even come to mind until late into the evening. I wrote them all down during a sleepless night.

I should have asked the hydrotherapy room attendant if the patients were kept in the tubs day and night. "No" would have been the right answer. They were taken out of the tubs at night, kept in leather restraints until the next morning, and then immersed once again. Did they eat? They were fed by the attendants. How did they go to the toilet? Once a day, temporarily placed in leather restraints, they were taken out of the tubs to sit on a toilet.

At the time of my tour of the hospital, pursuing my career decision to become a psychiatrist , I had just begun a three month Manteno Hospital stay. The year was 1956. Dr Nathan Apter, a psychoanalyst and professor of psychiatry at the University of Chicago, ran a research unit at Manteno, a mega state hospital located more than 50 miles from Chicago. And Apter had granted me a research assistant position. The pay was one hundred dollars a month plus room and board. Not very much, but the prospect of learning a great deal about schizophrenia made the job look attractive. Little did I know what I was in for, that living at Manteno for three months would change my life forever.

Few medical students, even those most interested in psychiatry, tried for the Manteno research assistant position. Manteno sounded like the kind of place that anyone in his right mind would want to stay away from. Yet there was something more to it, something strange. It was widely known that of those who did apply, even those from the top third of the class, Apter would reject almost all of them. Looking back years later, what had been a puzzle finally seemed to make more sense. Apter's unusually selective choices for the research assistant job probably had to do with how most of us thought about psychiatry at the time.

All of the medical students interested in the field of psychiatry envisioned themselves as psychoanalysts to be, sitting at the head end of a couch, listening to patients lying there, and telling us their problems. We saw ourselves occasionally making brilliant life altering interpretations based on what the patient had said. Psychiatry, psychoanalysis in particular, had a certain glamour. We read Freud's and other psychoanalyst's accounts of their work with patients. We were fascinated at what we were learning about how the human mind worked. Attached to our new understanding was this revolutionary therapeutic tool, psychoanalysis, that could be used to help people who had all kinds of mental conditions. Or so it seemed.

Enamored by psychoanalysis, most of us tried not to see that for the majority of patients our mentors' efforts at psychoanalytic treatment yielded little therapeutic success. Perhaps it was on this point that I differed from my peers. It was clearer to me than to many of the others that whatever we were doing in the name of psychiatric treatment at the University, psychoanalytically based or not, it wasn't at all adequate. It was a simple fact, clear enough even then for those willing to face up to it, that nothing much really worked.

During our six week rotation through the psychiatry inpatient service only those patients whose illnesses appeared relatively less severe, such as those suffering from moderate depression or anxiety, seemed to get any better. The majority of very sick patients, those overwhelmed by illnesses where a break with reality was the most prominent symptom, were sent off to Manteno State Hospital after a failed trial of treatment. There was a kind of invisible chute, the back door of the University psychiatric unit, that seemed to lead directly to Manteno.

To us medical students, Manteno was a very mysterious place. We knew that places like Manteno State Hospital existed all over the country, and that 800,000 such patients were kept in these places for indefinite periods of time. And the total population of these hospitals was rising at the rate of 50,000 patients per year! If you were a young person newly afflicted then by schizophrenia, we learned that you had a one third chance of making a complete recovery, even without treatment.Your recovery was called "spontaneous remission." As for the others, one third improved to some degree, though their lives were significantly impaired. The remaining third did not recover at all and went on to become progressively more demented.

Manteno's more than 8,000 patients were crammed into a space built to house 6,000 at the most. And there seemed to be no upper limit. Several times a week, sometimes almost daily, an unmarked blue bus would depart from some place in Chicago bearing a human cargo of twenty to forty newly court committed patients bound for Manteno. And the bus would return usually empty. It was a one way ride. If you got to Manteno, it almost always meant you weren't going anyplace again—ever!

As I look back,I can now make a good guess as to why Apter singled me out to become his research assistant, leaving my more brilliant classmates wondering why they hadn't been chosen. While I, like my peers enroute to a career in psychiatry, wanted to become a psychoanalyst, I had also become fascinated with the bizarre behavior and illogical speech of the few schizophrenic patients I had seen, and with the many schizophrenic patients I was reading about. And in my interview with Apter I couldn't help but talk of what little I knew about schizophrenia, and my fascination with the mystery of what must be going on. Of course I had explained that

I wanted to become a psychoanalyst. I could easily see myself seated at the head end of a psychoanalytic couch. That vision was clear. But the scene at Manteno, trying to treat very sick psychotic patients, that picture was a blank. It was almost inconceivable. Yet for me that scene was a magnet. What were all these schizophrenics really like? I knew that they seemed to be in another world, a very miserable one. Surely something had to be done to help them. Some of my reading had suggested that psychoanalysis could be adapted to a form where even schizophrenic patients might be helped. Working at Manteno, using some of these new techniques, might be my chance to help. And, of course, I needed to answer the driving question that repeated in my mind—what were all these schizophrenics like down deep? How did their minds really work? All this I explained to Apter. And he had listened.

Manteno itself was the repository of thousands of patients with schizophrenia, a sea of serious psychopathology where my full time presence could lead to learning far more than I ever could from reading books and papers in scientific journals. If I were chosen by Apter to go to Manteno, I would follow in the footsteps of some the great psychiatrists in history, Bleuler, Kraepelin, Arieti, and Freud, who had also spent periods of time working in mental hospitals. Their accounts of what they had seen was inspiring. Their efforts to understand the patients they were working with was exciting to me.

Whether it was my burning interest in schizophrenia or some other deciding factor, Apter picked me for the Manteno job, "to help" he had said. I don't know what I expected, but to say the least, when I got there, it was hardly what I could have ever imagined.

Two long lines of silent, disheveled, pajama clad patients were waiting for the electric shock treatments to begin. Dr Asher was standing before them, a small man with slicked down hair looking like a grinning ring master at a circus. Next to him on a small table was a little black box, approximately twelve inches square. From where I was standing, I could make out several dials and a button on top of the box. A wire connected the box to what looked like ice tongs that could be easily adjusted to fit the size of anyone's head. A hospital gurney stood next to Asher and his black box.

I had read something about electric shock treatment. The treatment had been based on the belief (later to be proven erroneous) that those who suffered from epilepsy never developed schizophrenia. Therefore it had seemed logical that artificially produced epileptic seizures might actually cure schizophrenia. The results of early trials had been significant, and within a decade electric shock treatments were being given all over the world for the treatment of schizophrenia and a wide variety of other psychiatric conditions as well. No one really understood how it all worked. Someone had characterized the use of electric shock treatments as "like kicking a Swiss watch".

Asher gave me a brief lecture about the shock treatment, his special area of expertise, how it worked for almost every condition, from alcoholism to adolescence, from schizophrenia to manic depressive illness, from depression to the ordinary nastiness of patients with character disorders. The current view, he said, was that it seemed fabulous for everything. He authoritatively explained that electric shock treatments worked by confusing people, and that this confusion enabled them to forget their troubles.

And it was quick and seemed very efficient. With his black box and the ice tongs applied to the temples, in an hour he could zap seventy to ninety patients. He once thought sixty was the max, but he had recently surpassed his old record. "It takes a system" he proudly explained. "Just watch this!"

At some silent signal that I missed, the first expressionless patient hopped onto the gurney like a well-trained seal. Then four other patients, two from each line, quickly moved forward and pulled up a sheet to cover the patient on the gurney. In unison they held the patient down by pulling tightly on the corners of the sheet. The moment the patient was securely in place, Dr Asher stepped forward, applying his ice tongs to the patient's head and pressing the button on the black box with the other hand.

A few seconds later I heard a surprisingly loud whoop, the sound coming from the patient on the gurney, his face now twisted into a hideous red mask. At the same time, his body arched against the gurney. Then after a few moments the rigid arch changed into a series of rhythmic jerks; large at first, then gradually dampening in intensity. During the whole process, the patient stopped breathing and turned blue from lack of oxygen. I wondered if he were ever going to breathe again. But the jerks finally stopped, and the patient took a big breath and began to look alive. A moment later he opened his eyes in a state of total confusion and stared blankly at Asher. Then upon Asher's signal, the gurney was whisked out of the room to return empty a few seconds later. To my amazement one of the four sheet holders then jumped onto the gurney to become the next patient to be subjected to the treatment. Her place as a holder was taken by another of the patients from one of the lines.

Asher said that holding the patient down reduced the likelihood of neck or back injuries, once common when patients were left to convulse without any attempt to dampen the intensity of their movements.

It was all as Asher had said. He clearly had a system for mass administration of electric shock treatment. And one after another the patients received a mini electro-cution as therapy for whatever their condition might have been.

I had never seen a *grand mal* epileptic seizure before this, and I was startled and more than a bit frightened by the first treatment.

Perhaps to counter my fear, I impulsively asked Asher if I could have one of the treatments "just to get an idea of what it is like." Asher seemed to give my request a moment of serious consideration. Obviously I had surprised him with the foolishness of what I was asking for. Finally he declined, commenting, "That isn't such a good idea." Instantly I realized that I had made an absurd request, and I felt like an idiot. I could envision the hospital superintendent, Dr Chermack, and Dr Apter hearing about my inane statement and having a good laugh. Apter might have second thoughts about having chosen me as a research assistant. This dreadful demonstration of my stupidity made me feel fragile and uncertain. I wondered what dumb thing I would do next. I resolved to try to at least appear a little more composed even though, inside, I was an agitated wreck.

"This here room is for colonic irrigations. High colonic irrigation is used to wash out the poisons that cause schizophrenia. We wash out the toxins, and patients get lots better." The attendant was nice to me, in sharp contrast to some I had met earlier in the day; but he was obviously confused as to what I was doing there. Clearly proud of his work, he was eager to explain it to me. He had total conviction that schizophrenia was an illness that could be washed away with the right series of ablutions.

The room itself contained a series of five tables, each with an assortment of various tubes, pipes and bags, all ready for use the next day, the attendant announced. An adjacent anteroom contained a few porcelain toilets. No one was being flushed at the time of my visit. I had missed the morning enemas. The attendant told me that the irrigation treatments were being given daily. The frequency of treatment for each patient was prescribed by the unit doctor and ranged from two to four times per week.

I wasn't disappointed at having missed the colonic treatments of the day. Even imagining a group of people simultaneously receiving mega-enemas and evacuating made me feel sick to my stomach.

The "Scotch Douche" room at Manteno looked like a parabolic cave lined with green tile. At one end of the room four high pressure fire hoses were securely attached to a metal pillar which ran from floor to ceiling. At the other end of the room was another floor to ceiling pillar. Here extremely violent patients were tethered to a metal post and sprayed by streams of water from the high-pressure hoses. The idea was that up to several hours of high pressure hosing would leave any violent patient exhausted and much more manageable. "It always works," the attendant said.

The door to the room burst open, admitting two burly attendants dragging a large man, thrashing and screaming, struggling against the straight jacket that bound his arms to his body. His wild kicks at the attendants didn't come close to landing. In almost no time at all, he was tightly secured to the metal post opposite the fire hoses. Aimed directly at him, the hoses were turned on full blast, and high pressure streams of water hit him from different angles. Assaulted by forceful torrents, he cursed for a moment or two and then began screaming and moaning. After a very long five minutes he slumped to the floor, a silent, immobilized rag doll.

This patient had committed the unpardonable sin of injuring an attendant. And according to the injured attendant's coworkers, he would have to pay a price for it. After a five minute interval, the hoses blasted him again.

"This is to get the devils and demons out of the patient's brain and keep them out," explained the 'Scotch Douche' attendant. In my head I knew I was witnessing torture, but there was nothing I could do. I was ashamed that I did not have the courage to demand that the hoses be turned off. Not that it would have done any good. And there was no one I could even tell about it. Apter and Dr Chermack must have known all about what was going on. It was just part of normal "treatment" at Manteno.

I asked what would happen to the patient once he was no longer possessed by demons? The attendant said he would be moved to the wet pack room.

The wet pack room was my next stop.

Earlier that year I had dutifully gone along with my medical school class to visit the Cook County Hospital morgue. Here on one table after another lay dead bodies of all ages, sizes, shapes, colors—the harvest of the Chicago streets for the previous night.

The "wet pack" room was almost like that. But the Cook County morgue had been brightly lit, filled with doctors and technicians all trying to figure out why each victim had died. Here the room was barely lit at all, and approximately fifteen blue-gray-looking pajama-clad men and women were strapped to tables with leather restraints. They all looked dead, but they were still alive. A group of three attendants, who no doubt didn't care if any of their patients lived or died, mechanically covered each patient's body with cold packs. The patients were then further covered over by the same gray canvas cloth I had seen earlier in the hydrotherapy room. I was told that the cold packs were changed every few hours. This was another form of treatment used to reduce violent be- havior. No attendant on duty at the time seemed to know why certain patients were given the cold pack treatment, while others were sent to the hydrotherapy tubs.

I was incredibly eager to leave this torture factory, to see some daylight and breathe some fresh air.

Most of the patient units at Manteno were two to a building. The outsides were uniform red brick one story structures. If one didn't know better, from outside Manteno looked like a lovely Midwest college campus. The insides of the buildings revealed a very different reality.

My tour of the hospital of horror had begun several hours earlier, when it was barely light. I wasn't the least bit sleepy that morning. In fact I was quite excited. I knew I was going to learn a lot on my tour. I couldn't have imagined what I was about to see.

The men's combative unit was at the top of my list. The name itself should have alerted me to something, but I didn't quite get it.

When I rang the bell of the building that housed the men's combative unit, I'd expected to be greeted by an attendant who would act as my friendly tour guide. Instead the person who answered was beefy, surly and nasty. "What the hell are you doing?" he asked. He didn't buy into my story that I was a research assistant on another unit, that I was there to get an idea of what the whole hospital was like. I then added that Dr Chermack had told me to visit this particular unit, and his stance suddenly changed. When he heard about Dr Chermack, he seemed to assume I was her spy, visiting to see if he and the other attendants were doing their jobs. He grudgingly agreed to let me in, but it wasn't much of a victory for me.

When he swung open the door, the stench of stale sweat was overpowering. That plus my first glance inside and I wanted to go no further. Before me were two hundred angry men, a swirling sea of gray clad creatures whose non-stop screaming and cursing was terrifying. My impulse was to excuse myself and run away, but it was too late—the door was closed and locked behind me. I was trapped!

"You could get hurt here," said the attendant. I was sure he was right. And my body automatically shifted into a primitive fight or flight status. I was hyper-alert, my heart beating fast. I could feel all the muscles of my body tensing, gearing up to protect myself when I was attacked. I could now see more clearly that as the patients milled around some would start hitting one another for no reason and then, most of the time, back off without any intervention. The attendants were a well trained team, and squads would occasionally fly off to break up the most egregious outbursts of violent behavior. About a dozen fights were going on in the room at any given time. As some would settle down, others would begin. "Mostly they don't get hurt too much," the attendant explained. I didn't see how that was possible. He then added in a matter of fact way that it was rare that someone was serious hurt, though there were occasional deaths. And some patients who demonstrated sustained violent behavior might be transferred to other units for "more intensive treatment."

The combative men's unit, like many of the units at Manteno, was a large gray warehouse, divided into thirds. The middle room was the day room. On either side were dormitory rooms with beds bolted to the floor in order to prevent their being used as battering rams. By day all of the patients were locked in the dayroom. There was no furniture because, "They will be throwing it at one another in no time."

A group of attendants began to usher me around the dayroom, acting as my human shield of body guards. And I needed them for sure! As we moved along, crazed screaming combatants would hurl themselves at us or swing at us. My cordon of attendants would expertly repel them, most assailants melting back into the crowd.

Guided by the attendants who really didn't want me there at all, I dutifully completed my tour of the unit. I couldn't wait to get out of there. Despite the world of violence around me, I escaped untouched. As I heard the door lock behind me, my heart was pounding, my own sweat pouring, and my chest felt tight. I felt lucky that I had survived.

What was I doing here at Manteno anyway? Was this all real? It was that odd detached feeling you only get when you are under high stress, the one where you stare out at a strange world through a thick glass window that isn't really there. You just aren't a part of the scene. But you are. I felt like I was very little and very helpless, much more like a lost little boy than a junior medical student. I tried to chalk it up to being scared. I had to pull myself together and go on. After all, I reasoned, could anything be as bad as the combative men's unit? But what if the answer were, "Yes?"

Having partially recovered, I moved on to the next place on my list, the women's geriatric unit, only a few buildings away. This time the locked door was opened by a more friendly attendant. He even smiled. As I stepped into what was usually the day room in other units, I was overwhelmed by the smell of urine and feces. There before me was a parking lot of beds, each occupied by a frail, obviously malnourished, elderly woman. Some were in restraints. Most were dressed in hospital gowns, although some had torn off their gowns and lay naked on their beds. Unearthly demented shrieks, cries, and groans made me feel that I was in the presence of alien creatures rather than human beings. These patients were still alive, but their souls seemingly had departed from what was left of their bodies.

As we toured the unit, the pleasant attendant told me in a very matter of fact way that all of these people were waiting to die, and that all would die fairly soon. There were deaths on the unit almost every day, and the same number on a men's geriatric unit as well. Probably one hundred patients at Manteno died each month. No one on the geriatric units ever got better. And no patient was ever transferred to a medical unit for treatment if his or her condition deteriorated. The attendant staff made some effort to clean the patients, change their linens and give them fluids—either water or a thick milk-like drink. The staff knew, and I soon figured it out, that these were token efforts at patient care.

One frail patient made a grimacing smile as we walked past her bed. She reached out to me with a tooth-pick thin hand. And I reflexively took her hand in mine. To my surprise she then clung to my hand with far more strength than I imagined she had in her whole body, as though thriving for a moment on the experience of human contact. Was this what she really needed? Had no one touched her in days, weeks, even months? Was she here at Manteno just because she was old and being thrown away? The attendant unpeeled her hand from mine, and we went on. My heart felt heavy as I thought about her. For a moment I wanted to go back and hold her hand. There was no way out and no comfort for her except to die.

When a few minutes later I looked back over my shoulder at the lovely red brick building I had just left, I couldn't believe what I had just seen inside. I felt terrible, overwhelmed with the realization that at least some of these elderly patients didn't belong there, that they were there merely because no one cared or because no one could figure out what else to do.

What happened when these patients died? I looked over to another building a few hundred yards away. Its fifty-foot smoke stack suggested that it must be a crematorium. I guessed that when patients died, social workers sent out notification letters. The families may have forgotten who the patients were, or perhaps had moved far away emotionally if not geographically. Probably most of the Notification of Death letters were returned to the hospital as undeliverable. While the patients had been alive, they were mere remnants of people. Once they died, they became names and numbers on a list filed someplace in a drawer that was never again opened; as though they had never existed.

Another red brick building on my list contained the insulin coma unit. The word, 'coma' summoned up instant apprehension. It was a word that commanded attention and respect. Everyone knew that 'coma' refers to a very serious medical state on the border of death. If you were comatose, you might very well die. If you came out of a comatose state, everyone was overjoyed, perhaps even thought it a miracle. But that wasn't the way things were at Manteno.

When I entered the insulin treatment unit, before me were twenty beds occupied by women in various stages of coma, all induced by injections of large doses of insulin given earlier in the morning. I had studied this procedure in a psychiatric textbook, but had never seen anyone in a coma before. Dr Lowell, the supervisor of the unit, was kind enough to teach me about it. She was one of the few Manteno medical staff members willing to talk to me. Yet for all her willingness to explain what was happening, it was not easy for me to concentrate. While she calmly described different coma levels, I was greatly distracted, since in the background I could see that many of the comatose patients were experiencing one epileptic seizure after another.

The seizures were the result of the injected insulin precipitously dropping patients' blood sugar levels to the point where, because their brains were deprived of adequate metabolic energy, they went into coma. What amazed me was that in any other setting, either coma or repeated epileptic seizures, called status epilepticus, was seen as an urgent medical emergency that demanded immediate, intensive medical treatment. Yet Lowell paid no attention to the nonstop perilous seizures going on around her.

Here at Manteno, I realized, these dangerous events were considered desirable. But in my mind it wasn't desirable at all. I didn't say a word. I knew that my screaming was really all in my head. It was all so backwards. Was I the one who was crazy? And when I talked, all that came out was a shaky-sounding question about the possibility that some patients in status epilepticus might die.

Lowell insisted, however, that there were very few deaths from the procedure: "Perhaps one-to-three percent," she said.

I was stunned. Lowell was calmly confirming my worst fears. How could a procedure with a one to three percent mortality rate be considered an acceptable medical practice? Later, in a psychiatric literature review, I would reconfirm this disturbing mortality rate.

If a patient did not become sufficiently comatose or failed to experience seizures, a higher dose of insulin was injected the following day. For young women with acute paranoid schizophrenia, Dr. Lowell explained, insulin coma was the treatment of choice. Many of this group responded dramatically. They became less paranoid and delusional; and over time, she emphasized, many returned to reality. Most patients received a series of fifty treatments. While she explained everything, I could only focus on the fact that these poor patients were having fifty brushes with death!

Some precautions were taken. An energetic nurse walked briskly around the unit, quickly and confidently shoving a large tube into the mouths and down into the stomachs of some of the comatose patients whom she had judged were seizing too much. She then poured a thick, syrupy fifty-percent glucose solution into a funnel at the upper end of the tube. After a few minutes,

the patient's epileptic seizures diminished in frequency and finally stopped. At the end of an hour
in coma, all patients were tubed and given the
syrupy solution to elevate their blood sugar levels.
I watched a few patients begin to sit up and stare
quietly around the room in a confused way. They
truly seemed as though revived from the dead. I
felt relieved. It was, indeed, like watching one of
those old zombie movies; only this time the movie
had come to life.

Dr. Lowell and I then walked into the catatonic
feeding room next to the insulin coma treatment
unit. Patients with catatonic schizophrenia were
stiff and mute. Some with catatonic schizophrenia
did not eat or drink. If left to nature, they would
die of dehydration or starvation. In the catatonic
feeding room I watched a nursing staff attendant
push a cart with a five-gallon jug full of a milky
fluid from one bed to another. Painfully thin, silent,
catatonic patients in various grotesque postures
lay in every bed; crumpled, emaciated manne-
quins each staring blankly into another world.

In a procedure similar to what I had observed
in the insulin coma unit, thick rubber tubes were
forced into each patient's stomach. The milky fluid
was poured into funnels at the top of the tubes. I
was happy to see that no one was drowning as a
result of an incorrectly placed tube pouring fluid

into a patient's lungs rather than into his or her stomach. After a feeding of only a few minutes the tube was withdrawn and the cart moved on to the next bed. Catatonic patients were fed twice daily. I left the unit wondering if each patient got a clean feeding tube or whether the same tube was used for everyone. Just the thought made my own stomach knot up.

Mentally ill patients with a concurrent diagnosis of tuberculosis were quarantined in their own special unit. By now I was exhausted, and the tuberculosis unit, thank goodness, was near the bottom of my list of units to visit.

What struck me at once was that the crowd of some one hundred patients milling around was very boisterous and active. I was told that many of the tuberculosis patients were receiving a new antituberculosis drug, Marsilid, which really seemed effective in arresting their lung disease. However, the drug also seemed to affect behavior. Patients who took Marsilid grew more alert, sleepless, irritable, happy, silly, and possibly more psychotic. As I walked through the unit, I observed people chattering at one another in happy nonsensical conversations. Some chattered at me and bounced away without expecting a response. It was just as well. I was feeling numb and energyless and couldn't answer anyway. I felt like I was attending a very noisy cocktail party where everyone else had had too much to drink.

The Marsilid this group of patients received to treat their tuberculosis was the first monoamine oxidase inhibitor drug in use, later to be recognized as a family of powerful antidepressants. But at that time we did not think much about antidepressant drugs. Using drugs to treat depression was a foreign concept to us, a minor problem, so it appeared, in comparison to the need to treat chronic schizophrenia.

There wasn't much left of me by the time I had completed my hospital of horrors tour. Yet there was to be almost no sleep for me that night as the visions of what I had seen kept replaying in my head. Until today I had been a normal student, half serious and half full of fun. After this day, the fun half part of me disappeared. This had truly been one of the most remarkable days of my life. I slowly walked back to my room in the medical staff building to rest and regroup. I had seen first hand what I could not have dreamed existed. It all felt unreal. Indeed, how had I gotten into this? Was it too late to get out? Somehow I had to tough it out.

Jim was a psychology grad student who worked part time at Manteno. He provided my transport to Manteno on Monday mornings and back to Chicago on Fridays. I liked him from the start. We could talk comfortably and freely, and I came to look forward to spending time with him. After becoming acquainted on that first day enroute to Manteno, I'd asked him to tell me about the hospital. He tried to give me an overall description, but I couldn't listen very closely. I heard something about 400 acres, some uniform style of colonial architecture, massive overcrowding. It was large, very large, he explained, a city onto itself, with its own power plant and laundry. There were many other hospitals almost like it all over the country. Years ago at Manteno they'd had a typhoid outbreak, and a number of people had died. But it was all cleaned up now. His words were drowned out by the song in my mind. Again and again I kept singing, "We're off on the road to Manteno!"

Of course the road to Manteno was a drive into another world. The University of Chicago was a medieval castle surrounded by the best and the worst of the twentieth century. To the East lay parks and modern high-rise apartments and Co-ops, all vying with one another to provide their occupants with the very best of views of Lake Michigan. On the other three sides the University was largely besieged by endless run- down neighborhoods barely one step above the nearby areas of actual slums.

That morning, on the road to Manteno, Jim and I drove forever through a world where everything was gray and black, the product of endless years of industrial pollution infiltrating every brick of the innumerable box-like, closely packed almost identical apartment buildings. Broken and tilted fences revealed yards full of rusty, windowless cars or unidentifiable junk. Beyond the decaying neighborhoods close to the University were the factory districts that seemingly manufactured soot as their principal product. After awhile the clusters of factories began to thin out as we came to the border of urban civilization. A few small houses here and there marked the rest of the trip. Occasionally we saw a farm house and some small fields. Wherever Manteno was located, it was in a different world from the one where I lived. More importantly, it was cut off from the world where we all lived; that seemed to be one of its primary purposes. To be sent to Manteno as a patient was indeed as though being exiled to another planet.

Every unit at Manteno was named after a famous psychiatrist. Except for Freud and a few others, most of the names were foreign to me. Dr Apter's research unit at Manteno was called Freud II. The title had made me smile, but nothing else about Manteno was the least bit funny.

On the day of my arrival at Manteno, I had met with the superintendent, Dr Chermack. She called me "Dr Widroe", an appellation that as a medical student I had never heard before. I had tried to explain that I wasn't a doctor yet, that I was really a student with very little experience in psychiatry. But she reassured me that my qualifications were more than adequate, that some of the other thirty doctors there at Manteno did not have licenses, many did not speak English, and a few might not even be real doctors at all. She needed help to deal with those 8,000 patients, and thirty doctors and thirty nurses didn't even come close to being an adequate number.

Freud II was to be my unit, she explained, adding I need not be worried that I would hurt someone. The eighty patients who lived on Freud II had been in the hospital for at least five years and the prospect of their ever improving or leaving the hospital was close to zero.

In my mind I was determined to prove her wrong. There had to be some way of helping at least some of them. I was sure that Apter would help me figure out what to do.

Manteno looked like a small city with more than one hundred buildings. Most were arranged in rows of identical H shaped structures set side by side along what could pass for city streets. Each half of the H shaped buildings held approximately two hundred patients (except for Freud II). The cross bar of the H was a dining area used sequentially by residents of each of the two units.

The units themselves were divided into two dormitories, each with multiple rows of metal beds. Once painted with cream colored enamel, they were now rusty and badly chipped. A single large day room lay in-between the dormitories. All of the rooms were totally gray, as though color were forbidden. The rooms had high ceilings. What windows there were hugged the ceilings. By day patients milled about the day rooms or sat in old wooden chairs, literally doing nothing except staring at blank walls or a single TV set somehow suspended from the ceiling. This was were truly one of the warehouses packed with human beings, all waiting for life to pass. Thus the majority of patients who lived on Freud II never left, and not only because they were locked in. The real prison did not turn out to be the walls and locked doors. The real prison was the nonstop nightmare of serious mental illness, a nightmare from which these patients could not wake up. Patients this sick had a total lack of motivation to ever leave.

Most of the Freud II patients were dressed in faded or gray clothing, giving the impression that they, like the walls, were colorless and lifeless. For the most part they were very quiet. Some were totally mute. None of the patients talked to one another. The only conversations were a few sentences exchanged between attendants, and if specifically questioned, an occasional short response from a patient.

Late in the day after my hospital tour when I got back to Freud II, I was emotionally drained. And I was incredibly relieved that my tour was over. Freud II, even though a part of Manteno, now looked great compared to what I had seen. For the first time, I had noticed the streams of light coming through the windows into the gray caverns of the warehouse that began to feel like my home. The Freud II patients, disheveled and mute as they were, suddenly appeared to be models of mental health who were being treated in a civilized, humane way. I began to experience warm feelings welling up inside of me alongside the pleasant realization that the Freud II patients now had become my patients. They needed my help and my protection from the gruesome torturers masking as treatment staff in other parts of the hospital. My efforts might actually make some difference in their lives. Not only was I going to protect them, I was going to help at least some of them to get well. I clung to this soothing feeling.

Eighty schizophrenic patients seemed way too many if I were to try some form of intensive psychotherapeutic approach to treatment. There just were not enough hours in the day to meet regularly with all of the patients. Besides that, a handful of the eighty were lobotomy victims. Apter regarded lobotomy as execution of the soul. These were truly hopeless cases, living robotic bodies without people inside.

Of the others I finally picked half a dozen whom I planned to work with almost daily in intensive psychotherapy. The rest of the eighty patients I did see briefly three times a week while I was on 'Doctor's Rounds', a medical school tradition consisting of a group of doctors, nurses and medical students moving from bed to bed interviewing or examining every patient on the unit. In this instance I was the only 'doctor', and my entourage consisted of one attendant and the Freud II social worker.

Apter visited every two weeks and headed the rounds group on the day of his visits. He was my mentor, a source of incredible information about all of the subtypes of schizophrenia, the clinical progression of events in the life of patients who were stricken by the illness, what to look for that marked change for the better, or for the worse. There seemed to be no end to his knowledge about treatment— good, bad, promising, futile. And I tried to absorb his every word. On the evenings after Apter's visits I did my best to record everything he had said. It was to become part of my Manteno diary.

The months at Manteno flew by. I recall the energy I spent meeting with each of my selected group of floridly psychotic patients day after day, trying to make some contact with them, to establish an alliance, to build a kind of platform from which to help them climb back into reality. I wanted to convince Gloria that she was more than a shit factory, and Tom that he wasn't responsible for single handedly keeping the earth from falling into the sun. I wanted Bill to make more sense when he talked, and I felt guilty that the only consequence of my efforts was his being transferred to the hydrotherapy unit because of his increased menacing behavior. All my efforts at psychotherapeutic treatment were to no avail. And as the futility of my efforts grew more apparent, I became more and more depressed and discouraged.

As I drove away from Manteno that very last time, I guessed that Manteno would never change except to house even more patients. There they were, all 8,000 very sick humans—some waiting to die, others just waiting—trapped forever in their private psychotic nightmares and imprisoned, perhaps forever, in the warehouses of Manteno State Hospital.

Happily for all of us, I was so very wrong. But from my vantage point at the time, I couldn't grasp that tremendous changes were about to occur, changes that would lead to the closure of most of the madhouses. It was only a few years later that the further development and wide-spread use of classical antipsychotic drugs such as Thorazine, Prolixin and Haldol, amongst many others, led to a precipitous drop in the number of state hospital patients. The new drugs, if used properly, could control, even erase, many of the schizophrenic symptoms. Once control of the illness was possible, it become conceivable to keep chronically ill patients in their communities. Within a few years the Manteno population dropped to 4000, plateaued for awhile, and then through death or transfer fell to zero. Throughout the whole country many hospitals like Manteno closed and were ultimately plowed under.

III. THE BEST OF THE MADHOUSE ERA

In 1956 psychiatric treatment wasn't all like the mad-house of Manteno. A few places like the Menninger Clinic or McLean Hospital were regarded as the premier hospitals in the country for the treatment of the men-tally ill. Most University medical schools and many general hospitals had psychiatric services. But these were generally looked down upon as ineffectual. In some, like the University of Chicago Clinics, psychiatry didn't even have the status to exist as its own department. It was considered a branch of the Department of Medicine, a branch barely tolerated by the rest of the medical school faculty.

Housed in a huge gray stone complex of connected buildings, the University Clinics were a dynamo for medical research, teaching, and treatment. The medical complex blended into the rest of the University, a world of towers, turrets, grand halls, libraries, classrooms, groined vaults and passageways – all built to emulate the 'Oxford medieval' style. The University buildings themselves appeared to exude the wisdom of the ages. And everyone at the Clinics – faculty, staff, students, and patients – regarded it as an honor just to be there to absorb something enriching, enlightening, and healing.

As a third year student, I rotated for three months through the University Clinic's psychiatric inpatient service. All medical students were mandated to have this exposure to patients sick enough to require psychiatric hospitalization. Most students hated psychiatry and regarded the psychiatric service as something they had to endure. For the few of us planning to go into psychiatry, the opportunity was heavenly.

Students were mostly present to observe. As far as being involved in the treatment of patients, our hands were tied. Yet while we were assigned to the inpatient psychiatric service, we did gain some limited experience simply by being around psychiatric patients and occasionally interviewing them.

"My problems are doors, locks, windows and walls. I don't know what to do about them. I think about them all of the time. How can you not think about them?"

Sarah, a nicely groomed young woman obviously in her last trimester of pregnancy, sat a few feet away from me in a small interview room.

I had never talked to a psychotic patient before. Yet just being in the presence of the florid psychopathology

I'd previously only read about made me almost euphoric. I was eager to say just the right thing and anxious that I might not. Needless to say, I tried to follow a standard memorized outline of the questions I was supposed to ask. But I found the patient's jumbled answers disconcerting and felt almost foolish as I doggedly pursued my script. Finally I asked Sarah what she was going to name her baby. Her shouted response, "I'm not pregnant!" startled me. Immediately I realized I had made some terrible mistake and was glad that no professor was in the room to have observed my blunder. As nicely as I could, I tried to point to the glaring reality. "It's all gas," she insisted, and refused to answer any more of my questions. She glared at me in angry silence for awhile, then walked out of the room.

I didn't have a clue what was wrong with Sara except that she seemed crazy. And that idea I had to keep to myself. I couldn't let the faculty know that I'd made such an unsophisticated unscientific diagnosis. I thumbed through my textbook of psychiatry and decided that, when asked, I'd answer that Sara suffered from either some form of schizophrenia or a type of obsessive compulsive disorder.

The inpatient psychiatric unit itself was in an L-shaped corridor with a walled off nursing station at the elbow of the L. Screened glass windows enabled the nursing staff to observe the unit. One half of the unit pretended to be an upscale hotel with elegant furnishings and richly carpeted floors. The recreation lounge on this unit was comfortable—even luxurious. This unlocked unit was intended to house those less troubled patients who supposedly would be comforted by their plush surroundings.

For the more disturbed patients, the other half of the L was locked and stark. The floors were linoleum tiles. The beds were cream colored plain metal hospital beds. There were no pictures on the walls. The unit was light, but there were almost no colors except for orange plastic chairs. All of the closed unit rooms were lockable—to be locked from the outside only. The closed unit also had two seclusion rooms behind heavy doors with small windows covered by a wire grate. Here the beds were bolted to the floor to prevent their being tipped, rammed or thrown by some superhuman mad-man. The locked unit lounge was filled with those standard orange plastic chairs plus a TV set anchored to the wall and ceiling. The face of the TV set was covered in screening wire to prevent it from being smashed by the more violent patients. It turned out to be a needless precaution. Years later we came to appreciate that, for mysterious reasons, TV sets are almost never damaged in psychiatric hospital lounges—even those units tenanted by the most paranoid and assaultive patients.

Patients could be interviewed in their rooms or in one of several interview rooms. And the patients were interviewed endlessly. They were interviewed by the assistant professors, the interns who rotated through the psychiatric service for a month, the social workers, the nursing staff, the occupational therapists, and finally even by the medical students. The interns might order various lab tests and psychological testing. As for the medical students, we were not permitted to order anything.

After all this evaluation over a ten-to-fourteen day period, each case was presented to the full professor or associate professor at a grand rounds or at a morning case conference. Patients were often briefly interviewed at these conferences. The professor finally gave his stamp of approval to the diagnosis or else suggested a better one. Only then was a treatment plan formulated and put into action.

During the evaluation period there was invariably little if any treatment. By faculty edict, there was supposed to have been no treatment at all. Occasionally, by accident or out of compassion some staff member secretly sidestepped the evaluation system. In theory, the premise for postponement of treatment during the evaluation period sounded fairly reasonable. We evaluators were not supposed to cloud the process of making the correct diagnosis by making apparently premature, haphazard attempts at treatment.

But there was a significant flaw in this system. Patients did not remain stable, unchanged specimens during the evaluation process. One forty-five year old engineer, Kenneth, was admitted to the inpatient unit after he loudly denounced several coworkers, claiming they were spying on his work and following him home. Although quite delusional, he was also perfectly lucid and coherent at the time of admission. But each day after he arrived at the hospital he grew more detached, withdrawn, confused and ill-kempt. Over a period of one week he became mute, incontinent, and stiff as a rod. Before our eyes he had developed catatonic schizophrenia and finally required tube feeding. A neurological work-up was undertaken to investigate the possibility of severe organic brain disease. None was found. After a few more weeks with no improvement, he was transferred to Manteno State Hospital for an indefinite period of care.

We painfully watched Kenneth deteriorate while we stood by doing nothing except 'evaluating'. My best friend, Josh, and I shared a sense of helplessness and frustration. Each of us felt there was something terribly wrong about doing nothing. The need for careful evaluation had a scientific ring to it. But on the medical or surgical services no one would have stood by watching while a patient's condition worsen. It seemed quite clear to us that delay in providing intensive psychiatric treatment was extremely harmful—especially in a psychiatric hospital where a patient was away from family, friends, surroundings and routines that may have been sustaining him. We saw that without treatment many patients tended to seriously decline. As they became worse, their ability to function at even the basic tasks of life often disappeared. By the time treatment got under way, the patients had often regressed so massively in their ability to perform the basic activities of daily living (such as showering or getting dressed) that the task of treatment had become Herculean. The absurdity of all this seemed blatantly clear to Josh and me, but no one would have listened to the opinions of mere medical students even if we'd had the courage to speak up.

Those patients admitted to the unlocked unit seemed altogether different. They all had become temporarily overwhelmed by easily identifiable stresses of life such as troubled marriages, jobs perceived as too demanding, or difficult children. Most of these patients were exempted from the teaching system and were designated as the private patients of the senior faculty. They were seen by their attending psychiatrists three or four times per week for psychotherapy or psychoanalytic sessions. No medical student was permitted to interact with these patients in any except the most superficial way lest we contaminate the treatment. The hospital staff was relegated to doing nothing more than providing clean linen and three average meals per day.

When we did interview patients on the psychiatric service, we were expected to follow a specific set of five basic simplified rules of psychotherapy; and we were eager to have simple simple guidelines, the more simple the better. Human behavior seemed so very complex. And five easy to learn lessons promised us a quick way to at least appear to act like psychiatrists.

Rule #1. Establish a doctor-patient rapport. That meant talking to patients in such a way that they began to trust you and saw you as someone who wanted to be of help. I liked this rule, and it quickly became embla-zoned in capital letters in my mind. Even to this very day I think this rule has paramount importance. Patients can not honestly confide in someone they do not trust.

Rule #2. Help patients clarify their thinking about problems in their lives. This often meant restating what the patients were saying, though in somewhat different words, or else just asking questions. I liked this rule, too. It sounded so easy. It also seemed to indicate to the patient that you were listening closely, and that you had an interest in his or her problems. It stimulated patients to talk more.

Rule #3. We were expected to take a passive stance. The intent of this rule was to let the patients do the talk-ing and come to their own conclusions instead of our pushing, advising, or preaching. The rule came from the psychoanalytic procedure of having patients free associate while lying on a couch. Even then I regarded this rule as unfortunate. In fact, I found it unbearable. I wanted results, and patients wanted results, and an active stance seemed the best way to get them. Patients always wanted information, and they wanted or needed direction. Often they were making very bad self-destructive decisions, and they needed active help to chart a different course. It was difficult, if not impos-sible, for me to shut up when the right advice often was so obvious. What I didn't understand at all was why it was so difficult for patients to accept constructive life altering counsel.

Rule #4. Make connective interpretations that would help patients understand how their current feelings, symptoms, or actions were products of unresolved problems of childhood. This was another derivative from psychoanalytic technique. It sounded wonderful! My fondest hope was that a patient would have a 'light bulb' turn on in his brain as he realized the truth of my brilliant insight connecting something happening now with something that had happened in the past. But I almost never saw the light bulb flash. I comforted myself that my apparent failure to produce results was only a product of my lack of experience. I wanted to believe that once I became more skilled as a psychiatrist, the light bulbs in the patient's mind would flash more often.

Rule #5. Try to identify our own feelings elicited by the patient and keep these emotions from having a negative effect on the treatment. I was puzzled about this rule at first. I had assumed that my role as a physician and psychiatrist would always remind me of how I was supposed to feel and behave. I thought I would easily be able to act from the position of being a benign white-coated helper. But it didn't take long to realize that different patients through their appearance, their statements, or their actions were going to elicit different feelings in me. A large muscular man shouting threats easily scared me, even if I was wearing a white coat that presumably marked me as a good guy who should not become an assault victim. Attractive women talking about their personal lives made me anxious and distracted me from the professional task I was attempting to pursue. No doubt I did have to contend with these feelings if I was going to be of help to anyone.

Following the rules seemed like good training. But apart from a small number of evaluation interviews, we had little opportunity to try them out. We were almost never allowed to act as therapists in any patient's treatment. Josh and I pushed and begged to have more active involvement in the treatment of any patients who might benefit from our inexperienced efforts. Our entreaties were generally ignored or rebuffed

But at times when a patient's treatment seemed to be going poorly, which was all too often, we were given a chance. For example, Karen, a middle-aged, obsessive junk collector had not responded at all to the program of treatment developed for her at grand rounds. Her home was packed floor to ceiling with newspapers, old paper bags, magazines, unopened mail, piles of clothing, and refuse. Josh, received special permission from a sympathetic faculty member, Phil Margolis, to accompany the patient, along with a social worker, to the patient's home in an attempt to give her the strength of will to throw things away. Josh had a talent for being loud, forceful and commanding, and yet kindly and supportive at the same time. As he urged Karen to fill boxes and bags for the refuse can, he made one psychoanalytic type of interpretation after another. "Come on, Karen! No one will die if you throw away those papers. No one will be hurt. You can do it, Karen!" The upshot was that a lot of stuff was tossed away. Yet Karen really did not change as result of the experience.

The frustration of our efforts at treatment was with us every day. Was this because we were so inexperienced and inept? Were our efforts the right efforts? Were our patients really untreatable?

But a few new and exciting things were starting to happen in the field of psychiatry.

Intravenous Ritalin was being tried as a treatment for depression in older people. Josh and I watched Phil Margolis slowly inject Ritalin into the arm of an older depressed man. After a series of injections the patient reported he felt no different. As far as we could observe, he did not seem to act any different either. We were very disappointed.

While this attempt seemed to have failed, Phil explained that another new technique, slowly injected sodium amytal could have dramatic therapeutic consequences. Totally mute catatonic patients became able to talk for an hour or two. Patients with amnesia remembered who they were and what had happened to them. Other patients with hysterical paralysis discarded their wheel chairs as they began to walk again. And there was the new French sleep treatment.

Magic! It had been like magic. And a ray of hope!

Joseph was an ox-like 275 pound six- foot-five-inch engineer. For a few days prior to his admission to the University psychiatric service he had become increasingly suspicious, argumentative, and confused; his anger finally escalating until he assaulted one of his coworkers for no apparent reason. The police were called. After a brief struggle, he was subdued, restrained, and brought to the University hospital psychiatric unit. At the time he was admitted he was hollering and threatening. His ravings made no sense whatever. He pulled and jerked against the leather restraints that bound his wrists and ankles, and it seemed he would burst out at any moment to commit mayhem. Just being around him was frightening.

Yet that was my medical student assignment. I was to work with the nursing staff as an extra pair of hands to help in his management. I was given an eight hour shift, midnight to 8a.m., to be with him in his locked seclusion room. Apart from the bed where he lay restrained, the room was devoid of any other piece of furniture except for the chair where I sat and watched. While Joseph slept, I tried to read my psychiatric textbook. My text confirmed my suspicion that Joseph suffered from acute schizophrenia. How exciting, although frightening, to see the illness in real life.

Here in the seclusion room Joseph was given a series of injections of Thorazine, a promising new medication, also known as the French sleep treatment. After several shots Joseph did fall asleep. From then on he was aroused every six hours, carefully taken out of his ankle and waist restraints, toileted, and given fluids along with more Thorazine in a liquid form. He was then returned to a totally restrained position on his bed.

One week later the Thorazine was discontinued. Over a 24 hour period Joseph became increasingly alert. He even began to talk to those of us who took care of him. The magic that I saw was incredible. The monster was gone. The man who awoke was pleasant, sensitive and polite. He made sense when he talked. His grasp of reality seemed to parallel my own, except that he had no idea what had happened to him.

If someone as sick as Joseph could improve so dramatically, couldn't everyone? Was schizophrenia really so incurable?

We took most of our questions to Phil. He had recognized that Josh and I were not just the ordinary, uninterested medical students who suffered a forced rotation through the psychiatric service. We were clearly intensely unhappy with the magnitude of our ignorance. Phil proved to be kind and approachable and gave us lots of time for discussion. We could question, protest, speculate, and create. Yet Phil had only a few of the answers to our questions. Topics we discussed with him ranged from which patients had the best prognosis if given insulin coma treatment (young women with acute paranoid schizophrenia) to what had Freud really meant in *Mourning and Melancholia* about depression being inwardly directed aggression. Not that it really mattered. There was no way that we, as medical students, were ever going to get the opportunity to try out any new or old techniques. All of our treatment orders were "proposed orders" which everyone ignored — it was all pretend!

The psychiatric service at the University did not seem to have a good track record. Most patients did not get well. And our self-esteem as an institution was very poor. When we were able to transfer one unresponsive patient to the Menninger Clinic, we regarded it as an honor. We envisioned Menninger as a magical hospital, like Oz in a cornfield. We believed that at Menninger, and a few other high power hospitals in different parts of the country, psychiatric cures were the rule; cures that could never come to pass on our unit. For us Menninger embodied our fantasy. It gave us hope that cure was possible. But, like most fantasies, the reality was very different. Despite its great image, Menninger was just another psychiatric hospital. We later discovered that even Menninger had a chute to its own overcrowded state hospital.

That we were a poor demoralized psychiatric service was really no different from any business that proves unprofitable. As with an athletic team with a poor track record of wins and losses, we'd had way too many losses. Far too few of our patients were getting well. Looking back, we clearly did not have the tools to help people get well. Our cabinet of curative agents was almost barren. We were not sure what really worked and what did not. Some patients got better, and we liked to think it had something to do with our efforts. Or was the improvement merely the mystery we called spontaneous remission, like recovering from a bad cold?

My interest in actually living at Manteno had been sparked by Richard Siegler, a medical student one year ahead of me. He had a perspective on many aspects of life, and an outlook I had never before encountered in a young person. He told me that most students were idle dreamers who had brilliant coffee shop ideas but little if any capacity for follow through. "If you want to play the piano," he asserted, "don't sit around complaining about your parents never having given you lessons when you were six years old. Do something!" So why should I complain about the inadequacy of my training in psychiatry at the University? Living at Manteno for me was doing something.

IV. THE CHUTE TO INSANITY

As we drove up to Manteno that first day I was struck that even up close the hospital still looked like a college campus. But there were no crowds of students moving in different directions or just milling around—only an occasional person in the distance, like a dot on the horizon. Where was everyone, I wondered. Where were the 8,000 patients?

Then I saw a line of dots moving from behind a building. At first the line appeared as a column of ants—all moving along toward some unknown destination. As they grew closer, I realized I was looking at shabby gray people shuffling along in single file linked by an invisible chain. An attendant stood alongside, his voice the whip that urged his charges to move along just a little faster. Apart from the crack of his voice, there was no sound. No patient said anything or seemed to look at anything. Even as I grew close to the silent column, no one looked over at me or in any way acknowledged that I existed. They shuffled on and left me alone.

Where had they come from? Where they were going? Were they typical of everyone here? What was the matter with them? Why didn't they talk to one another? I knew I would soon learn the answers to my questions.

The doctors who worked here at Manteno all seemed to hide from one another. Even the medical staff dining room was very quiet. All the doctors ate meals together, seated at several long tables. Altogether I counted close to thirty doctors; most dressed in shabby suits with frayed shirts and ugly ties. Verbal exchanges were few. I tried to be sociable, but no one really wanted to talk with me. It wasn't as if they did not like me in particular. Everyone seemed to be hiding from something or someone in the real world; and for various reasons no one wanted to expose himself or reveal his true identity.

Once there was an unexpected stir of conversation in the medical staff dining room. This came following the sudden disappearance of Dr S. who had stolen off without notice into the night. The story was that Dr. S. had a serious drug addiction problem, which was why he had been working at Manteno in the first place. The circumstances of his leaving were unclear, since no one had talked to him or observed his departure. No one really knew him, either. Rumor had it that he had fled with a supply of medication he'd stolen from his unit. Another story was that his cravings had become so intense that he had fled to seek drugs outside of the hospital, perhaps from his old dealers. A real mystery. But by the next meal it was as though Dr. S. had never existed.

I learned that hundreds of higher functioning patients held volunteer jobs maintaining the grounds, working in the laundry, the kitchens, the maintenance department and in housekeeping. I was told that these jobs were considered privileges.

I had a quick internal debate. Were the patient jobs really privileges? Perhaps some of the patients were doing what they had to do in order to get out of the hospital, a kind of penal servitude. Or they were earning good behavior points, trying to look good before their doctors as a way of bringing them closer to freedom. On the other hand maybe the jobs enabled patients to escape the boredom of sitting around a hospital ward day after day with nothing to do. The work might even be therapeutic. It might help people, I thought, by giving them more structure to each day; perhaps give them a sense of achievement, which, in turn, could increase self-esteem and self-confidence.

At my first medical staff lunch I got to meet Dr. Gallagher. Since he worked on my unit some of the time, I hoped I could befriend him. But he could not look straight at me for more than an instant. I tried to talk to him. I told him who I was and what I hoped to do and to learn. The talk was very one-sided. He never once asked me a single question or commented on any subject I had introduced. Actually he appeared pained at every question I asked. He looked red in the face as he squeezed out short, single-sentence answers to my questions. He had an apartment on the same floor as my dorm room. I would visit his apartment only once during my three month stay at Manteno, and not by invitation. The occasion was my need for an answer to some procedural question. My visit with him was literally a minute's duration. He reluctantly ushered me in and then practically pushed me out. Gallagher's apartment was remarkably clean and extremely well-ordered, not like a place where anyone actually lived. Despite my staying at Manteno for months, I rarely saw Dr. Gallagher. According to the Freud II staff he visited my unit occasionally, but always after 5 p.m., when I was certain to be gone. It was never clear why he wanted to keep away from me. Was it something I had said or something I was doing that he didn't like? Or was it all his problem?

It seemed that almost all of the attendants who took care of patients at Manteno State Hospital hated their work. Most had migrated to Manteno from the southern part of Illinois or from Kentucky following the closure of a number of coal mines where they'd worked for many years. Pay at the hospital was poor; but the workers had little education and few skills, if any, to make them eligible to compete for better paying jobs in Chicago. Most lived on the hospital grounds. Others lived nearby in the small town of Manteno. All in all these people struck me as bitter about life and showed no apparent concern about patient care. Like the patients, they too were trapped indefinitely at Manteno State Hospital. There were almost no younger people. Those few younger people who were there had only come to Manteno because their parents worked there. All had hopes of a better life elsewhere. But the majority of the attendants here were middle aged, and for them Manteno must surely have seemed like the end of the line.

The attendants' training was "on the job", and minimal. They performed in a mechanical way. They treated the patients as objects. Not people. Were they cruel? Although I could never prove anything and never saw any overt displays of cruelty, I was certain that at times the attendants were physically abusive to patients. An old truism related to me by Apter during one of his visits was, "When you come to the unit in the morning and see that two or three patients have become catatonic over the previous twenty four hours, it means that a patient has been beaten by the staff the night before." The inference was that patients who were catatonic were "scared stiff." An act of violence on a unit could lead to the development of a catatonic state not only in the patient who had been beaten but in others, too, who felt threatened as they witnessed a beating.

All of the buildings at Manteno State Hospital were named after famous psychiatrists. No one was testing me, but I was ashamed that I recognized only a few of the names. At the same time I was immensely pleased and even proud that my unit was called Freud II. The other names all related to ineffective treatments of the past. But the name Freud stood for those psychoanalytic techniques that I felt certain were going to evolve into the major effective treatments for all mental illness. The Freud building was identical to the vast majority of the buildings on the campus—another beautiful red brick building with surrounding lawns and lovely, well-kept plantings now slightly brown with the winter season. But it turned out that my unit and almost all of the beautiful red brick buildings on the campus were like stage sets. Unlocking the front door and entering the unit you stepped from color and sunshine into a gray dusty world inhabited by strange, bewildered shadows of people.

The H shaped floor plan of Freud I and Freud II was divided into two identical units. Freud II itself contained three large warehouse like rooms—a dormitory for forty or more women, a dormitory for forty or more men, and a connecting common room. All of the rooms had ceilings at least fifteen to twenty feet high, dwarfing the crowd of inmates who wandered below. Tall windows admitted a good deal of light to the dormitory rooms, but even the sunshine failed to bring warmth or light to the patients. The common room had fewer windows and seemed dim even on sunny days. Everything was gray. The floors were covered with darker linoleum. The dormitories contained nothing but rows of solid metal beds whose chipped, cream-colored paint announced years of neglect. The main feature of the common room was the TV set, anchored to the ceiling and wall, as it was at the university clinic, but with no protective screening here. Many plain badly scratched and worn wooden chairs were generally aiming toward the TV screen. Except for meal times, when it would be turned off to induce patients to go to the dining area, the TV set was on all day long, performing before a captive distracted audience.

Freud II patients ate together in the cafeteria-styled eating unit that formed the cross bar of the building's H layout. The patients from the other half of the building, called Freud I, used the same dining area just before it was used by the Freud II patients. From time to time the staff doled out faded but clean clothing to patients. The clothing distribution followed some sort of schedule, though I never clearly understood it. Some of the clothing belonged to the individual patients. The rest came from a community supply. The unit was so self-contained that it was possible for a patient never to leave. The majority never did.

Patients were not permitted to spend daytime hours in the dormitories, and during the day they milled about in the common room or sat quietly in front of the TV set. They seemed unaware and unconcerned about what program they were watching, whether a game show advertising shampoo or a sermon threatening death if the viewers did not reform their ways. Other patients in the day room, often smelling of urine, stood in bizarre postures like statues and did not move for hours on end. There were no conversations between patients. Attendants occasionally addressed patients regarding where to go or what to do, but there was no reaching out to engage patients as people with feelings or needs. Occasionally one attendant addressed another, briefly, usually about the work at hand. This was the type of warehouse from which the term "warehousing patients" had originated.

While Esther was designated as the Freud II secretary, in fact she was the executive who ran the unit. She looked like a middle-aged, somewhat overweight housewife. She dealt with the never-ending stream of paper that came to and left the unit. She maintained the medical records of our patients and knew all of the medical record deficiencies. She was keenly aware of which charts did not have the required annual psychiatric evaluations and which ones did not have quarterly progress notes. She knew which patients had privileges allowing them to attend occupational therapy at another building on the campus. She could list from memory those who could take attended walks, who could be unattended, which patients had work privileges and what those work privileges actually were. Although not a clinician, she knew the patients who warranted privileges if they did not already have them. She would periodically leave notes for Dr. Gallegher telling him what management orders he should write. As far as I knew, he always followed her instructions.

Esther was positive, energetic, organized, and cheerful. The grim atmosphere at the hospital did not seem to have any negative effect on her mood. Perhaps living off campus with her family enabled her to remain calm and pleasant. Needless to say, Esther, the ward executive, instantly became my mentor. It was Esther who tried to answer all of my questions. When after my first few days on Freud II, Esther complained that most of the patients needed psychiatric evaluations and progress notes, I was only too happy to comply. I was thrilled at the prospect of making some positive contribution. By her example, Esther taught me the importance of having solid support staff in running any enterprise.

Art was the unit social worker. What was left of his hair was prematurely gray. His rasping voice slowly conveyed his detailed thoughts. He always looked fatigued. He was a kind and wonderful fellow; it went without saying that he had to be kindly in order to tolerate the frustrations of his work. The many furrows on his forehead told of the burden he bore, the weight of eighty-five mentally ill patients' insoluble problems. Part of his job was to write lengthy reports to different agencies and to answer the all-too-infrequent family letters of inquiry. For many patients such letters were nonexistent since they had no contact with the world outside of Manteno. After awhile, families seemed to give up. Being a patient at Manteno often meant being cut off forever from the rest of the world. Seeing myself as apart from the patients, I could only thank my lucky stars that such a fate hadn't befallen me. At other times, seeing what was all around me, I was just too sad for the patients to even think about my own happiness.

The rest of the Freud II staff consisted of Dr. Gallegher, whose presence was only an elusive shadow, and the sullen attendants who were ill-suited, unwilling, uneducated and without leadership to provide more than a semblance of patient care.

The only other person who should be mentioned was a mystery nurse whom I never saw. He visited the unit twice daily to dispense medication to those few patients for whom it had been ordered. Most patients were not receiving medication, both a sign of the times and a reflection of the sense of futility that pervaded the unit. Why bother giving these patients medication when they were hopeless anyway?

That first day I arrived on Freud II, I made efforts to smile at the patients around me. But I was too nervous to try to talk to them. No one smiled back, and no one talked to me or even asked me for a cigarette. In that era the asking for cigarettes or lights provided a universal framework for social discourse. It was an easy way to meet people—except here at Manteno it didn't work.

I was exhausted that night, but in spite of my fatigue I could not get to sleep. Everything was so new and strange to me. I lay in bed seeing in my mind all that had happened that day — from the drive to the hospital to the meeting with Dr. Chermack to my first visit to Freud II. At the dinner table I had wanted to talk to anyone about my first day at work. I wanted to talk to the other doctors, but their detached glare put me off. Each seemed preoccupied with his own thoughts. The somber group of taciturn doctors did not talk to me or even to one another. It was easy to feel isolated, and I felt very much alone. I got out of bed and read sections of Bleuler's book, *Dementia Praecox*, to try to make better sense out of what I had seen and was about to see. Somewhere in the middle of the night my tired mind finally wandered off from *Dementia Praecox* into a series of troubled dreams.

V. WHAT AM I
SUPPOSED TO FIX?

Prior to my coming to Manteno Apter had told me that I was to help out; but he had not been specific. Perhaps, overwhelmed with anxiety in Apter's presence, I hadn't listened closely enough to my charge. On my arrival Dr. Chermack had called me "Dr. Widroe" and had also said I was there to help. On the other hand, apart from welcoming me to the hospital and assigning me to Freud II, she hadn't told me what I was supposed to be doing there. Dr. Gallegher, who wanted nothing to do with me, certainly didn't tell me, either. So there I was without the slightest idea of what I was supposed to be doing.

Looking around the unit did not help clarify my charge. Nothing seemed to need doing except for curing the patients, and no one seemed especially intent on such a formidable task. Between Dr. Gallegher, Esther, Art, the mystery nurse and the attendants, the unit appeared to be taking care of itself in fulfilling its essential work. Its mission was to warehouse patients for an indeterminate period of time. The unit did not actually require my help to perform what seemed to be its most essential function.

After first coming to Manteno, filled with energy and enthusiasm to do something, it took me a few days to figure out that no one was going to tell me what I was supposed to do. Because Esther did not scare me the way Apter did, I appealed to her for help. "What have other medical students done here in the past? What did Apter want done?" Esther answered that she had not seen another medical student in over a year. She did recall that medical students who had been there in previous years didn't seem to do much of anything.

The thing that prevented me from asking Apter directly what I was supposed to do came from typical medical student insecurity. No medical student feels secure that he is going to actually complete medical school. When we first assembled as freshman, we were told that we had been chosen very carefully, and that we would have every bit of help that we needed in order to graduate from medical school. But there really was no help. The only help I can recall was the vague assurance that, unlike many other medical schools, our medical school had no formula for weeding out a set percentage of students by the time of entry into the junior year.

Most medical students only asked questions to which they already knew the answers, doing so with the intent of looking good to the faculty.

And that was my approach to Apter. I listened carefully. I studied a lot on the nights before his visits, and I knew a good deal about what I was asking before I asked. To ask Apter what I was supposed to do, I thought, would be casting a spotlight on myself as some fool who did not belong in medical school.

Esther had complained that the medical records for the patients on Freud II were in very poor condition. Most lacked any recent annual psychological status evaluation. Every three to six months Dr Gallegher would write very brief progress notes such as, " No change." This lack of change might have been true, but it was insufficient to constitute what needed to go into a decent medical record. An acceptable medical record required some substantive information about what a patient had been doing and even some semblance of a psychological status examination. Relieved to have been given some well-defined task, I resolved that the least I could do was to interview all of the patients and update the medical records in a proper fashion. Whoever would read them in the future, I didn't know. I suspected that no one ever would look at them except to see that they were there. Despite my concerns about the fate of any medical record entry that I might make, I knew that solid medical records are a critical part of good patient care. To the limited extent of improving the medical records,

I was going to make a contribution here at Freud II. I also would have something respectable and acceptable to report to Apter should he ever ask what I was doing. He never did ask. When I finally did tell him, he didn't seem the least bit concerned. He acted like he hadn't heard me.

The rest of my charge was really up to me. I would get to try what I'd wanted to do so desperately. I would treat some of the Freud II patients, even though they were considered to be hopeless cases. That treatment had to be some version of psychoanalysis that would work with schizophrenics. I didn't quite know what I was going to do, but I knew that I would figure it out as I went along.

Esther and Art shared an office adjacent to the day room. We decided that my interview room would be the linen room next to Esther and Art's office.

I had a table and two chairs moved into the linen room. I mentally erased the floor to ceiling shelves full of off-white, grey or badly faded clothing. I now thought of the linen room as my own psychotherapy office. The table was placed between the two chairs. The patient's chair was to be close to the door that exited into the day room. I was not sure who was going to be more scared in the therapy sessions — me or the patients. But I wanted to be protected by the table as a barrier, and I wanted the patients to feel that they could easily escape into the day room if they felt uncomfortable during our therapy sessions.

I hadn't forgotten my tour of the hospital. I had felt bewildered and overwhelmed for days afterward, as though I were in a bizarre dream. Yet despite the horrible things I had seen being done to human beings for their presumed betterment, my fear had been tempered by my disbelief. On that tour I was an anesthetized viewer, almost a tourist or visitor numbly looking at phantoms doing curious, unimaginable things. That special shocking day all I had had to do was float from one weird scene to another.

Everything would be different now. As I settled into what I envisioned as my real work in life, I began to experience a new set of feelings. At first it was curiosity about my charge, my responsibility, my duties. It became tension and nervousness ultimately blossoming into real fear with sweating palms, tightness in my chest and light headedness. These were symptoms of my fear of interacting with my own seriously ill patients in a direct and hopefully therapeutic way. They were all so ill and their behavior so surreal, that I didn't have a clue as to how to relate to them, and I was scared. I feared I might fail.

I had not been prepared for this. All the interview techniques and theories about what we were supposed to do that I had memorized back at the University now seemed totally inappropriate. But I needed to learn to be around these sick people. I needed to learn to talk to them. Somehow I had to figure out how to reach into their psychotic worlds and find out who they were and what they were. I was now being called upon to perform and felt like I was on stage at a piano recital before a huge audience. It was kind of an honor and a great opportunity to be on stage, except that in this scenario I had no idea at all about how to play the piano.

Art, always trying to be helpful, suggested we try to have a large mid-morning community meeting in the day room. I jumped at his idea. I invited Art to help me run the group. I thought I would learn how to talk to the patients if I followed Art's example. The attendants were puzzled about what we were doing. They dutifully pushed together a circle of about thirty of the badly scratched and worn dark-brown wooden chairs. A number of patients were invited, cajoled, and herded into the area and commanded to sit in the chairs in the circle.

I tried to start the meeting. "I am Dr. Widroe. I am going to be here on the unit for the next three months, and I want to get to know all of you. Can you tell me your names? " There was silence. No one told me anything. I repeated myself two or three times. Still silence.

The community meeting never happened. It never happened because no one was capable of being a part of a community. Gathering the patients for any event outside of mealtime or bedtime was like trying to organize a swarm of mosquitoes or flies. A few patients sat down on the wooden chairs as directed. Some who had sat down then promptly popped up and wandered off. Others came close to the chairs, eyed them suspiciously and continued to stand. A few more sat down minutes later. Of those who sat down, many had their eyes pointed toward the now blank TV screen. Were they still seeing pictures that I couldn't see? Even when I gave up and announced that the meeting was over, no one seemed to notice.

I retreated to the staff office adjacent to the day room. Esther and Art both sensed my feelings of failure and helplessness and tried to comfort me. They both said it would take some time, that I should try again the following day. But I knew instinctively that they were wrong. Nothing would be any different if we tried to have a community meeting the next day. Besides time was not a positive factor for me. I had only a limited period of time at Manteno in which to try to help someone to feel better.

I then came up with a different approach. There had been some precedent for all of the patients to sit next to their beds when medications were delivered to those for whom they had been prescribed. I decided to use this already programmed event to try to talk to at least some if not most of the patients. The next morning while the patients sat waiting for medications to be brought to them and before they came out into the day room, I walked from bed to bed accompanied by a friendly attendant. The attendant would tell me a few things about each patient before I tried to speak with him or her. This was to be my version of the University Clinics doctor's bedside rounds .

I felt tense and scared— fearful I would say something so stupid that the one attendant who accompanied me would recognize I was an ignorant imposter. Of course, I realized, in fact I was an imposter. I had never done this before. I wasn't a real doctor. I had tagged along on doctor's rounds at the University, but only as the most junior of a large entourage of white-coated ducklings headed by a professor. This time I was the head of my own mini-entourage consisting of one attendant, and I was about to interview patients who probably could not tolerate an interview. My concert performance was about to begin, and I felt like I didn't know the least thing about what I was supposed to do or how I was supposed to perform or even what the program was.

I tried to keep in mind the number one rule for conducting psychiatric interviews, the rule I really liked.

Basic Rule #1. Establish a doctor-patient rapport. It didn't just happen by itself. I had to talk to the patients. I had to act as though they were my patients, and I was there to take care of them. Maybe then I could build some kind of doctor-patient rapport. My goal was to help my patients move from total alienation to a state of trust.

Even though I could recite the other four basic rules governing student behavior in psychotherapy sessions, the only other one that seemed to have any relevance at all was:

Basic Rule #5. Evaluate how I felt about each patient. What were my feelings? That one was easy. I felt very scared – even even before seeing the first patient.

I walked up to the first bed. Ann, probably in her mid thirties, wore a stained and faded long sleeve striped jersey and a sack like skirt, both faded veterans of countless washings. "I'm Dr. Widroe," I said, trying to sound friendly yet professional at the same time.

"And I always mind my own business unless an enemy attacks me," she responded.

I felt totally lost. I did not have a clue as to how to respond. I knew I was being warned, and that I needed to be very careful in what I said. I dropped to my list of emergency questions, the ones you ask when you don't have anything else to say. "How are you sleeping?"

"I went to the dentist because I don't feel well."

"What's the trouble?" At least I could comment with a question relevant to what she was saying.

"I don't know," she answered.

"Do you have pain in your mouth?"

"Yes." Did this mean she had an abscessed tooth, or that she had a deep-seated unconscious problem stemming from infancy that had led to her developing schizophrenia?

"And what does the pain make you think of?" Could I help her make a connection between mouth pain and other fundamental issues in her life? But she did not answer. And I felt humiliated because my question sounded so stupid. I didn't know what else to say, and I stopped the interview. I walked away in the direction of the next bed. I envisioned a frowning Dr. Apter standing behind the attendant. Both gave me a failing grade in psychiatry.

Perhaps I had given up too quickly. The interaction had been poor. I had failed to establish even a semblance of a therapeutic alliance with Ann. On the other hand, nothing terrible had happened. And Ann had talked back to me. After a pause of a few seconds, I changed my mind. I concluded that my first interaction with a schizophrenic patient here on Freud II had been pretty successful. I had actually talked to a schizophrenic patient who, in a strange way, had talked back to me.

Betty looked thin and taut, her face frozen in a fierce grimace. She stood next to her bed staring off into space, rhythmically rocking back and forth. She did not respond to my questions at all. Just before I tried to talk to Betty, the attendant told me that Betty had strangled, dismembered and then boiled parts of her two small children. Once here at the hospital she had assaulted and seriously injured another patient. The hospital's response to her homicidal behavior had been to have her lobotomized. The rocking person standing silently before me was a post-lobotomized version of the Betty who used to be so violent and unpredictable. She had been someone I would not have dared to be near. While I talked to Betty, I regarded her as hopeless because she had been lobotomized. I envisioned lobotomy as severing the frontal lobes away from the rest of the brain. What was left of the person was a robot-like shell. Betty seemed to fit my preconception that lobotomy was really the execution of the soul.

Pearl did not look at me. I tried to be friendly and engaging. "Hi Pearl, I'm Dr Widroe. How are you feeling today?" But she did not answer any of my questions. Her mouth was grimacing as if sucking or chewing. She had a growth of facial hair not quite thick enough to be called a beard. She was constantly moving her tongue in her mouth. She responded to the attendant's direction to stand up or sit down. Apart from her mouth movements, she did not move. When I think back to Pearl, I am reminded that involuntary mouth movements occurred in schizophrenic patients long before the widespread use of antipsychotic drugs, now regarded as the villains in producing involuntary movements, a condition currently termed tardive dyskinesia. I instinctively knew that Pearl was too difficult a case for me; that I would never get her to talk to me and would never be able to help her. I hated to give up so easily, but Pearl was in another galaxy.

Gail appeared slovenly and dirty, and emitted a most foul odor. I wondered whether she had ever been given a shower. She spent most of her time sleeping in a fetal position in a chair. At irregular intervals she would make loud nonverbal cries. She often called out when she had to urinate and would wet herself if she were not led to the toilet immediately. Gail did not answer any of my questions either. By now I was getting used to the nonresponse type of response, and I no longer regarded each patient's failure to talk to me as the result of something I was doing wrong.

Time seemed to stand still as I went from bed to bed, trying again and again to reach out into the psychotic worlds of my patients and make some kind of contact—even a touch by eye contact or any response of a few words or sentences. No matter that the glance was fleeting, or that the words or sentences didn't make sense. And on occasion I did get some kind of response that made a modicum of sense. By the time I got to the men's dormitory, I was feeling more comfortable and more confident. I didn't think I had done anything too stupid. And I was starting to focus on observing the patients rather than being preoccupied with my own insecurity and fear.

Clarence presented the rare picture of being extra neat, well groomed and precise. He sat motionless, and his face was blank. While he spoke spontaneously and without prompting or questioning, his voice was flat in tone. The attendant told me that Clarence was improving.

"I was sick. I did not know which way to turn. I was confused. The pills help. My stomach was rotten. Good bowel movements get rid of the rotten stuff. The food is wonderful. My stomach is very small."

It was clear even to me that Clarence had a thought process disorder. His thinking did not make sense from sentence to sentence. He was also delusional with a number of distorted ideas about his body. But at least he seemed like he was someone I could talk to in therapy sessions. How exciting! Perhaps I could help Clarence.

Leo, a rugged looking man about age fifty, rose and extended his hand. He tried to answer my questions. At times his answers were almost related to what I was asking.

Leo opened the interview. "This is a great hospital," he declared, telling me that it was "Margaret Hospital." He knew it was winter because the weather was cold. He knew the year but not the month. He knew he was sick, and he liked being at the hospital. Beyond that his thinking jumped all over from sentence to sentence, and I couldn't understand what he was trying to say.

David looked like a teenager from afar; but up close I knew he was in his forties. There was something about the relaxed muscles of his face that made him seem much younger. He gave me my first exposure to 'word salad,' his thinking so scattered that he was talking in barely related single words and phrases. He also had 'echolalia' in which words or phrases almost rhyme.

"I don't know, ko, corn. I can't hear you, mother, Mary , fairy, God. God Damn! man, plan, asshole, dirty. Dirty flirty girls..."

I asked a few of my standard questions about how he was sleeping and how he was eating. His answers were not even remotely related to the questions. I wondered how I could connect with a patient like this. I could not see even the beginning of the doctor-patient rapport.

And I crossed his name off my ever shorter list of those I thought I could help.

I crossed many names off my list that day. I felt so ill-equipped and inadequate to be able to help most of the patients I had interviewed. I wasn't sure why names remained on my list. But I knew it had something to do with there being some thread of contact, perhaps ever so slight, that nonetheless gave me hope. Was it a smile? Was it a verbal response of any kind whether it be a short phrase or even a warning to stay away?

That evening in my room my mind was racing with exciting replays of my encounters with patients. Enthusiasm had replaced anxiety. My concern with being a medical student pretending to be a doctor had disappeared after half an hour of doctors' rounds. My new concern, more formidable, was my frustration at trying to develop relationships with people who not only didn't speak my language but who were in a whole different world. Different worlds might be more accurate, because each patient lived in his own universe. I wrote in my diary, as I did on numerous other undistracted evenings, recording what I had seen, what I had read, and to a lesser degree what I thought about it all. I tried to prepare myself for the next day. I scheduled the patients I planned to interview. I reviewed my goals. I wrote about what progress, if any, my patients might be making.

On Friday afternoons I talked nonstop to Jim Sachs as we drove back to Chicago for the weekends. I must have driven him crazy. But he tolerated me fairly well, and he tried to respond when I gave him an opening.

"If we were going to help them, we had to get through to them," I chattered. What was the key to talking to schizophrenics? Wasn't catatonia amazing? How could people assume rigid statue-like postures for hours on end day after day? Were they really scared stiff? Or were they so fearful of the delusional consequences of moving that they did not dare to move? How could people really hear voices talking when there was no one really there? Were the voices like the voices of real people talking in the room, or were they like the thoughts anyone has in his head except at higher volume? How did it work? Wasn't Jim curious (as I was) as to what the voices said? How loud were they? Were they all bad voices? Were any of them good voices? Did they ever stop? Did they ever change? Were they men or women? Did the patient know whose voices they were? Were they the voices of people they had known earlier in their lives?"

Jim did make some attempts to answer. During these days Jim was the only person I could openly talk to about my experiences at Manteno. I was disappointed that he seemed to have a less intense interest than I did. But then Jim did not live at the hospital. He did not have a unit of patients like the eighty-five patients who had now become my world twenty-four hours a day. He knew in general what went on at the hospital, but did not see it close up; and so Jim was much more distant from the world of severe psychotic illness than I was.

Nonetheless my own excitement seemed to pump Jim up each time we chatted. We kept talking about how to make the hospital better. We discussed simple ideas such as insisting that all patients who were not bedridden have attended walks around the hospital grounds. We had more imaginative ideas like firing all the nihilistic attendants and replacing them with armies of college students or college graduates who themselves were enthusiastic about life and really wanted to help people.

Most of my waking and sometimes my sleeping existence was filled with Manteno thoughts and feelings, yet I tried to have fun on weekends away. Sometimes I was successful. More often I was not. My review of what I had written in my diary the previous week seemed to take up a lot of my weekend time. But by Monday I was recharged, ready to take on the challenge of my plans for Freud II for the following week.

VI. THE FIGHT TO RESCUE SICK MINDS

By the beginning of the second week it was becoming increasingly clear that what I understood to be conventional psychotherapeutic techniques needed major revision for the treatment of chronic psychotic patients. Rule #1 about establishing a doctor-patient rapport still made wonderful sense; but the rule itself sounded grossly inappropriate for me at Manteno. The rule seemed like an attempt to describe normal nonpsychotic doctor-patient behavior to a spectator. But at Manteno that kind of relationship couldn't exist. It made far better sense if the rule were restated—changed to "establishing a therapeutic alliance." The change made the therapist focus on hope and treatment and getting on the patient's side fighting against the enemy of schizophrenic illness. Following this restated rule seemed challenging, but at least possible.

Rule #2 had been an attempt to help the patient focus on important problems and to think of these problems more clearly. How could this be done when a patient's thinking did not follow the usual laws of syntax and logic? Schizophrenic patients frequently couldn't focus on anything. Trying to make reasonable connections for someone with schizophrenia was like trying to nail Jell-O to a wall.

Rule #3 stated that the therapist was supposed to take a passive stance. What a joke! This rule bore no relation to reality whatever. Therapist passivity at Manteno would have as much impact on a patient as a speck of dust floating in the room.

Rule #4 needed to be revised. How could you make meaningful interpretations to patients with chronic schizophrenia? It might be one thing to tell someone who was not psychotic that he was depressed because he felt angry with his father. But how could you help a schizophrenic patient make sense out of such an interpretation? Even if the interpretation were heard, it would just slip away into the other globs of scattered thinking.

Rule #5, trying to keep track of how I felt in the presence of the patient always seemed to have value. I discovered that I could use that awareness. For example, when I talked to a particular patient, if I became uncertain or afraid, I could end the session. When I felt too interested or concerned, I could ask myself why I was more worried about George as opposed to Roger. I could then review whether my excessive concern was leading me to say the wrong things or making me spend more time with George than might be good for him. As I spent more time with patients, I found that my sensitivity grew, and I could make better and better judgments about what to say or do. But I would not fully evaluate my global emotional response to what I was trying to do until my days at Manteno were almost over.

The only formal attempt to teach any of the Manteno medical staff anything at all came at Apter's case conferences every two weeks. While the doctors' attendance at the conferences was mandatory, I often wondered if anyone besides Dr. Chermack and me was listening or even awake. Apter's teaching seemed to have a central theme. There were both physical and psychological causes of schizophrenia. Certain unconscious factors contributed to schizophrenia more than others. Apter also felt that some particular factors led to treatable, as opposed to irreversible, schizophrenia. These unconscious factors all stemmed from unresolved problems that had occurred early in life – most often in infancy. Under stress, later in life, the patient would manifest the symptoms of schizophrenic illness.

The treatment suggested by this conceptual framework was that psychotherapy must help patients deal with unconscious conflicts from early childhood – as though the core issue in schizophrenia had been a mother's feeding techniques, her attitudes, her stress level, or her very presence or reliability. Maternal abandonment or hostile attitudes were considered critical factors in traumatizing an infant; matters which, years later, could lead to a schizophrenic breakdown.

Excited by this background of psychoanalytic thinking, I felt encouraged to try out some of these newer psychotherapeutic techniques in treating chronic schizophrenia. While I had decided to focus my efforts on a handful of patients, I didn't want to neglect the other patients on my unit. Bedside rounds three days per week enabled me to observe and to interact briefly with each patient. I would then write progress notes into each patient's medical record. I could learn a good deal more about the phenomena of severe mental illness and progressively refine my interviewing techniques. These efforts could help me grow new skills for developing therapeutic alliances even with very difficult, negative and unwilling patients.

And that was what happened. Week by week I became more able to elicit answers to my questions and in turn to become more attuned to degrees of variation in a patient's thought process disorder or grasp of reality. I learned that some apparently reasonable patients would drift in their thinking with subtle shifts occurring from paragraph to paragraph. Sometimes it took listening to several paragraphs before I realized that a particular patient was not really making sense. Other patients shifted subjects from sentence to sentence. Still others 'scattered' from phrase to phrase or even word to word, the word salad I had only read about before I came to Manteno.

Patients taught me a lot about auditory hallucinations and the questions I needed to ask. How much of
the time did they hear the voices? All of the time? Half
the time? Every day? Was it a particular time of the day?
Only occasionally? How loud were the voices? Were they
louder, softer, or the same volume as my voice? What
did they say? Did they tell the patient to do things? What
things? Did they command the patient to harm himself?
Or to harm others? Did the patient ever do what the
voices commanded them to do? Sometimes they did
obey the commands, and the consequences of what
they did might be very serious. They might even jump
in front of moving cars, or try to harm themselves in a
multitude of ways. Were the voices critical? (They usually
were.) Or were they kind voices? (They rarely were.) Did
the voices belong to anyone the patient knew or had
ever known? Was it always the same voice? Did they
upset the patient?

Patients also taught me about visual hallucinations.
What did they see? Were they just fleeting shadows,
or were they substantive images? Were the visions like
dreams? Were they distortions of things that were real,
such as shadows becoming people? How often? Did
they see things more in the mornings, afternoons or evenings? Or did they just appear at any time without being
related to anything? Were they terrible? Did they scare
the patient? Were they like bugs, snakes, spiders, goril-
las? Or were they more like whole elaborate scenes –
for example, Christ climbing down from his cross? If they

saw people, did they recognize the people? Did they see and hear things at the same time, or were the visions quiet?

The differences in the answers to these questions from session to session became a measure of the severity of the patient's illness. They provided a critical, sensitive tool to use in measuring whether patients were becoming better or getting worse. Awareness of even nuances of change could lead to significant treatment plan changes by the psychiatrist.

I don't remember how I picked the patients I was hoping to cure. As I review my Manteno diary, I do not see specific criteria that I may have employed. I don't even see that I had selected a set number of patients. Some are mentioned in the diary much more often than others. I presume I had more interest and spent more time talking with them. No doubt my criteria included the patient's ability and willingness to talk, the absence of lobotomy (which I, like Apter, regarded as signifying that there was no prospect for recovery), and whether the patient seemed to like me or wanted to talk to me.

Armed with my enthusiasm, a rapidly developing skill at psychiatric interviews, and a smattering of knowledge, I charged into the asylum.

Over a period of months my efforts had mixed results at best. Bill was one of the patients upon whom my efforts seemed to make some impact. It seemed that week by week he had come to talk more, even though a lot of what he was saying didn't make much sense.

One day Bill was markedly agitated. He walked around the day room accosting anyone who crossed his path—patients, attendants and me. When he would approach anyone, he would threaten loudly with a barrage of angry word salad. His agitation was apparent in the volume of his voice, his excited shrill tone, and his choice of words suggesting or threatening physical violence. He grasped my tie, but he did not pull it. He responded to my questions; yet all his answers concerned beating, fornication, spying, and reporting to the police.

That evening, because it was feared that he might harm someone or himself, the attendants had him transferred to the hydrotherapy unit.

The next morning I went to visit Bill while he was in hydrotherapy. His head stuck up through the gray canvas that covered the hydrotherapy tub.

Bill: "Don't love me. I'm sorry I hurt you. I got crazy a little bit. I'll mind my business if you mind yours. You go too fast. I know you now. Don't mean to offend you, but I know about you. I got trouble just like you. I'm more here than you think. The silly way I talk helps me get by in this world. I like you. You think fast. I was punished for pleasure. I'm afraid of getting hurt. I sort of suffer. You are in my power. I like this world here, mind my own business, jerk off. When I was a kid, I'd go with the nicest people.

If I told you, I'd cry. You'd hurt me. I act dumb, but I'm crazy. Now I want to be left alone. I know who you are."

When I told Apter about Bill, he had said, " We have to tell all young residents in psychiatry not to try to cure schizophrenia in six months. Schizophrenic patients cannot tolerate intimate interpersonal relationships without great anxiety and probably the need to withdraw further or at least become very disturbed. If they could tolerate interpersonal relationships, they would not be schizophrenic."

While I was flattered that Apter considered me at the same educational level as a psychiatric resident, he was underscoring what I already knew. My efforts to treat Bill had been successful only to the extent that he had become threatening, agitated and possibly violent. I had left Bill in a worse state than when I had started my attempt to treat him. My attempt to cure had failed badly, and I felt miserably guilty that I had not done a better job. What I should have done better, I did not know.

Bill was right when he said he knew who I was. I was just a wild-eyed, well-intended, over-enthusiastic medical student trying to do the impossible.

VII. DOWN AND DEFEATED

During my last few weeks at Manteno the weather was turning bad. The sky became grayer and the cold more penetrating. At first I felt more tired in the mornings, a fatigue that became nonstop. For awhile I thought I had the flu. I was barely aware that I had begun to leave Freud II an hour earlier than usual. And I seemed to be losing interest in the patients. It grew difficult to concentrate. My efforts to talk with patients lost the energy that characterized most of my earlier interactions. I noticed that I did not think of the Freud II patients as 'my patients' anymore. That, in itself, seemed strange. In the evenings I paged through a few escapist novels instead of the books on psychiatry that had been my daily fare. My entries into the diary became shorter and shorter. After awhile it seemed as though I had nothing else to say, and I didn't care whether I said anything or not. Finally I stopped writing altogether.

For reasons I would come to understand only later, I decided to have a closer look at the occupational therapy service. Rather than take a tour, I thought it would be interesting to examine the service from a patient's perspective. When those Freud II patients for whom occupational therapy had been prescribed lined up to march off to the occupational therapy building, I got in line with them and shuffled right along. I became one more dot in the ant column of patients moving slowly and silently from one building to another. To an outsider I appeared like the other ants except that I wore a white coat instead of the shabby gray clothing worn by the other patients. Inside my head I forgot that I was wearing a white coat. The same invisible chain that shackled the patients to one another now had come to bind me as well.

Once we had arrived at the occupational therapy art shop, I sat at a long table along with twenty to thirty other patients. A staff person walked around the room giving soft spoken encouragement to those apparently willing and able to listen. Whether any of them talked to me, I don't even remember.

The patients were as silent as ever; a few of them working quietly at a number of different arts and crafts projects. I knew I couldn't draw, but I remembered modeling animals in clay while I was in grade school. So today it would be clay.The clay in my fingers felt oddly comforting, and I began to make an abstract clay sculpture about six inches tall. Within a few minutes I forgot about my plan to watch other patients using occupational therapy as a means of treatment. I became preoccupied with my clay sculpture and the good feeling that my own occupational therapy produced inside me. For a few minutes I felt moderately guilty that in an attempt to escape from my own unhappy feelings I was deserting my job as a healer of patients. Then the guilt melted away. Nothing other than sculpting seemed to matter, and for a short time it helped me feel better. I went back to occupational therapy on a number of days intent on to completing my piece. I felt mesmerized, now driven by an intense wish to do something positive.

Of course at the time it did not actually dawn on me that I was depressed. Like many who are depressed, I had no awareness that this was clinical depression and not the sadness that is part of the vicissitudes of day to day life. Depression was the name of the illness from which I was now suffering. And in occupational therapy I had become unknowingly engaged in my own treatment.

I still have that piece of abstract clay sculpture. While it appears to have some human features, it is ugly and forbidding. Its geometric curves, sharply cut planes and negative volumes are devoid of any human warmth. The cold and expressionless form reveals only how miserable I felt. Nonetheless, producing this odd piece of sculpture gave me a modicum of comfort at a time when I very much needed to be comforted and when little else seemed to help.

I spent more time in my room mulling over my many defeats. None of my patients had been cured. No one was even any better. A few patients had appeared to improve for a few hours or at most a few days and then were worse again. At best, they had become more upset and agitated than they had been before I attempted to treat them. Any degree of improvement had to be measured in very modest terms. For Harriet, improvement meant her talking more, even if only for a day. For Sam, it meant his transient resolution to get a job. For Bill it meant that his word salad level of thinking improved to become short and scattered sentences with more meaningful content. For Keith, improvement meant a single amytal interview that enabled him to take part in a one-hour chat. But for each patient, even these miniscule gains had rapidly disappeared. And Bill had ended up in a hydrotherapy tub.

At first all I felt was a sense of failure and futility. I had not helped anyone. I blamed myself for failing, after telling these patients that I could help them. But occasionally my thinking shifted away from self-recrimination. I began to have another kind of obsessive thought. Instead of repeatedly asking what I had done wrong, I asked myself what I had done right. What had led to even the most transient of gains? Apart from the intravenous amytal for Keith, whatever prompted change seemed totally mysterious. It did not seem to be the psychoanalytic interpretations suggested by Apter or Rosen and other psychoanalysts. I had tried these techniques repeatedly with at least a dozen patients. Unlike the reports in Rosen's book I could never connect any subsequent behavior change with my efforts. It seemed more likely that my patients' fleeting changes were related to the amount of attention that they received. My insistence and my urgency were a constant factor. I envisioned myself jumping up and down and screaming loudly at someone who was totally deaf. Even the very psychotic patients could not ignore me. It was my energy directed at the patients that somehow had rocked the boat of their psychotic worlds. Of course I was unhappy that some of them responded to this invasion of their psychotic space by becoming more agitated. Even more important, it took so many days and so many hours just to bring about a transient change. How could anyone effectively cure a chronic schizophrenic patient with psychotherapy alone? What hope was there for the hundreds of thousands of schizophrenic patients in all the Manteno look-alike psychiatric hospitals across the whole country?

On one of our Monday morning commutes to Manteno, Jim told me about a full professor in the department of philosophy at the University of Chicago who had a serious alcohol problem. One evening in an intoxicated state he had smashed out a number of plate glass store front windows along 57th street, a few blocks from the campus. The administration had placed him on administrative leave and urged that he seek treatment. Instead he had opted for a six-month period of self imposed penance by exiling himself to Manteno. But he had not come as a patient. He had begun work as an attendant.

"Wow, that is unbelievable!" was all I could say. I resolved to find the professor and to try to talk to him. Because he had such a unique profile, it took only a few questions of inquiry at the administration office to locate him. I cautiously and respectfully asked him if we might meet. He was amenable to the idea, and soon we began a series of late afternoon walks when his work schedule permitted.

I don't remember what Hugh looked like. But he seemed to exude a comforting glow that I could almost see. While Hugh was a warm person, he never talked about himself. And out of respect for his privacy and dignity I didn't ask him why he was there. He seemed to assume that I knew. He was just there at Manteno on leave from the University. He was there for awhile, doing work on one of the units. To me, Hugh was a genius. But what else should I have expected from a full professor in the Department of Philosophy? He was willing and able to talk about anything. Some of the time we actually did talk about Plato and Aristotle. But for the most part we talked about the hospital and its place in society and how it helped society avoid a problem it felt helpless to face. We talked of the impact of the hospital on the personalities and souls of the unfortunate patients housed there.

One evening as a line of silent patients shuffled past us, we walked side by side, more intent on talking than on getting anyplace. The two of us might as well have been walking on the University of Chicago campus. " Psychiatry is a very inexact science," Hugh said. "All applied sciences are like that. They have little, if any, claim to clear and exact truth. They are always in a state of flux even here at Manteno. While we cannot see the change from day to day, it is in a state of flux here as well." His ability to frame even the most painful and distressing reality in the perspective of a philosophical framework always surprised me. I recognized the shadows of Plato's cave somewhere in back of what he was saying. I wanted to believe him. I sought clarification of what he had said. I longed to learn some tiny fraction of what he knew. And he was kind enough to indulge my questioning.

Hugh came to be the person at Manteno in whom I could totally confide. I was certain that he would understand everything I was saying. He knew first hand and perhaps appreciated even more than I did what I was talking about. I told him about my hopes on first arriving at the hospital, and how those hopes had become translated into plans. I told him about my treatment efforts. I confessed to my failures and my resulting unhappiness. No one was cured. No one was really improving. It was as though I had never been there. My only lasting mark had been an updating of the Freud II patients' medical records.

Hugh listened in a kind and tolerant manner. He then gave me not one but two pearls of wisdom, each of which seemed like an incredible gift. The first pearl was, "Is this your whole life? This is but a second in your life, just as it is a second in my life. If you have lost any seconds from your life by being here, and I doubt that you really have lost anything, the seconds are few and should only be weighed against the hours ahead." I felt honored that the seconds of my life were being measured by the same clock that measured the seconds of his life.

The second pearl was, "You must make your work give you what you demand of it." I didn't understand him at first. He seemed to sense my puzzlement, and he explained further. "You have demanded something of your work that it could not provide. And you have not fully appreciated what it could provide and actually has provided. You have gained something incredibly valuable in all that you have learned."

I heard him clearly and realized his comments were extremely important even if I didn't fully understand them fully at the moment. Later that evening I wrote it all down in my diary so that I wouldn't forget any scrap of what he had said. His very words were treasures, never to be forgotten. I knew he was right. Yet knowing he was right, at least then, did not have an impact on the heavy weight I was carrying or on my sense of futility and failure.

A few weeks later it was all over. As we drove away from the hospital campus for the last time, Manteno looked the same as it always did. Even from afar I knew that Keith was still stiff and mute. Jenny was still a shit factory, and Zeke was still struggling to prevent the earth from falling into the sun. It seemed to me that it would always be this way. I doubted that Manteno would ever change.

No one could have guessed that within thirty years, as a result of the findings of a Governor's investigatory blue ribbon panel, many years after my three month stay, Manteno State Hospital would be closed forever. But in 1956 when I was there, the only certain change of which I was aware was the change that had taken place within myself. In three months I had aged ten years. The fun part of my life as a student had given way to the serious and determined preparation for my life's work.

VIII. A NEW ERA BEGINS

"Look to your left. Now look to your right. Next year those people won't be here!" We all believed legends about other medical schools where the incoming class had been warned from day one that if they didn't perform as well or better than their peers, they were out for good. They were out of medical school and probably enroute to some totally different kind of life than the medical career they had envisioned. As orienting freshmen, we had been assured by the dean of students that our school was different, and that the faculty were there to help us. All of them, we were told, wanted us to succeed. But we weren't that naïve. We knew the claim of faculty concern wasn't true at all. Faculty concerns were limited to their own research projects. A student might come to faculty attention only if he or she were willing to work on a faculty member's research project for no or minimal pay. We knew that if someone faltered, dropped out, or was asked to leave, that others were in the wings waiting to transfer in from who knew where if only given the opportunity.

It had been difficult enough to gain admission to medical school, each of us triumphing over huge numbers of other highly qualified candidates. It was as trying and highly competitive then, just as it is today. Pre-med students could be scheming and vicious. My girl friend, Peggy, a biology major setting the world afire with near perfect grades in a premed course, was offered a bribe by a group of premed students to stop ruining the grading curve. They envisioned that her excellent performance would undermine their grades and destroy their whole lives. Those who finally were admitted to medical school were bright, tough, and highly driven. But admission to medical school carried no guarantee of success.

We justifiably all carried a kind of survival paranoia that had some basis in reality. Everyone feared that saying the wrong thing, doing the wrong thing—no matter how innocent or insignificant, might be misinterpreted by any faculty member as sufficient grounds for us to be dismissed. Our hard fought pursuit of a medical career could just that easily be aborted.

Our fears were amplified when from time to time a member of the class actually disappeared. Nothing about it was ever announced. We were left only with rumors which served to heighten our fears. Sometimes the reason for the disappearance was obvious. One student committed suicide. We felt bad for him, and recalled that he had been a very likeable fellow. Another had been arrested for counterfeiting, an incredible act of folly! For the rest of us these seemed easily avoidable problems. Far more scary were stories of others who had been tossed out of medical school for reasons that didn't make good sense. In my own class there were a few such casualties. It defied all reason that a student was let go presumably because he had told a patient his blood type? If so minor a transgression led to expulsion, what trivial self-destructive sin might be inadvertently committed by any of the rest of us? Clearly an apparently innocent act, benignly intended, could lead to personal disaster.

As students at the University of Chicago medical school, our role in patient care had been all pretend. We were merely a very busy group of white-coated imposters, poor actors pretending to be doctors. Following our carefully memorized scripts we visited live patients with all too real problems, live patients who mostly knew who we were and who put up with us as part of the price of being treated, they hoped, by famous and apparently omniscient professors of medicine. Our written patient evaluations and proposed orders for patient care were merely teaching devices, stripped from a patient's medical record and shredded the moment each patient was discharged from the hospital.

None of what we did had any consequence in real life, and patients were protected from our well intended but often ignorant recommendations. On rare occasions a student might come up with an accurate patient diagnosis that no one at some higher level in the academic hierarchy had considered. While such individual brilliance merited a gold star often leading to an A grade in the course, it usually earned the undying animosity of the jealous and embarrassed resident or intern who had blown the correct diagnosis. For a medical student to pull off such a glorious performance was exceptional, and these enviable instances were few and far between. I was never so fortunate. I was just one of the non-descript medical students somewhere in the middle of the pack, trotting along, hoping I could make it to the finish line of graduation.

Needless to say, completion of medical school is an incredible relief to all medical students. The dean of admissions, Dr Simmons, had casually whispered the great news of my impending graduation when I accidently backed into him at the University bookstore. "Widroe, you are going to make it through. The committee has decided that you will graduate!" Hearing these shockingly wonderful words, no matter in what setting or how informally they were delivered, triggered a euphoric rush in my head. Suddenly I felt flushed and weak. While I didn't actually fall to my knees, I felt weak-kneed and actually tottering. Leaning heavily against a book counter, I somehow mumbled my thanks along with something stupid to the effect that I was going to make the committee proud of their decision.

Even as the words left my lips, I wanted to pull them all back. I feared that I had made some horrendous error, a gaffe with far reaching consequences. Because I had said the wrong thing, the committee members just might change their minds. The formal letter announcing my impending graduation might never come. But the committee decision for me to graduate was final, and, as the dean had promised, in 1957 I did matriculate from medical school. From there I went on to begin a one year general internship at Mount Zion Hospital in San Francisco.

In marked contrast to life as a medical student, internship meant real responsibility for patient care under the supervision of knowledgeable physicians whose patients we tended. We all worked long and hard, but always with the idea that our efforts were helpful, necessary and fully appreciated. We rotated through a number of different services, primarily medicine, surgery, and obstetrics and gynecology. At Mount Zion the interns and residents even ran an indigent clinic complete with house calls. We loved what we were doing, although it meant sleeping very little the every other night that we were on call. As interns our skills and confidence as doctors grew exponentially. My own self image changed dramatically during that internship year. White coat or not, until then I'd always felt that I was a fake, an imposter, a college student posing as a doctor. Now over the months I came to believe in my rapidly developing skills and actually to feel that I was a real doctor, a new self image that carried with it a sense of serious responsibility. When people looked in my direction and called out 'Doctor,' I no longer turned around to see who the real doctor was. I came to automatically assume that they were actually talking to me. And as a bona fide doctor, unrelated to how I was addressed, I became comfortable making decisions about diagnosis and treatment. With increasing skill as a medical practitioner came a growing awareness that my medical training, which I had once considered an obstacle course prerequisite to becoming a psychiatrist, would serve me well in treating psychiatric patients. Nonetheless I also more keenly understood that despite all of my reading and the Manteno State Hospital experience, I knew very little about psychiatry.

IX. TREATMENT AT LAST

Even with full awareness and a serious fear of the prospective consequences of my ignorance, in 1958, when
I entered my first year of psychiatric residency training at
San Francisco General Hospital, I could sense that I was
very different from the other first year residents. None of
the others had had any experience like my months at
Manteno State Hospital. None had observed and tasted
the horrific pain of psychotic illness and the frustration of
trying to rescue patients from a nightmare from which
they could not awaken. The other residents had not seen
large numbers of disturbed psychotic patients before. To
them schizophrenia, manic depressive illness, and obsessive compulsive disorder had been names attached to
text book descriptions rather than to live patients. They
were still like college kids, more interested in having a
good time than in serious business. In its unique way,
despite all of the pain and frustration I had endured in

my zealous efforts to treat people who at the time were untreatable, Manteno had prepared me well to begin my intensive psychiatric training.

Like most county hospitals in big cities, San Francisco General seemed to dominate the entire neighborhood. Walking from one end of the ugly multi-building hospital campus to the other was like taking a hike in an area totally devoid of attractive scenery. There was nothing for miles that anyone would want to look at—only things to look away from. No two buildings matched. None of the architecture displayed any feature that made viewing the buildings either pleasurable or memorable. There were no green spaces. Only asphalt and concrete parking lots separated the buildings from one another. There was nothing to distract us young doctors from focusing our thoughts on anything except patient care.

The San Francisco General psychiatric service was housed in a hulking five-story red brick warehouse-like building directly across the street from the emergency room. The psychiatry building contained four inpatient units—separate evaluation units for men and women and two acute treatment units all located on its upper floors. The first floor housed support services with offices for the medical director and her assistant, social services, clerical staff, an on the scene courtroom for commitment proceedings, and other administrative offices.

The floor plan of each unit was very different from my recollection of the Freud II layout at Manteno. The San Francisco General psychiatric units were T-shaped with a large dormitory and several seclusion rooms at the top of the T. Patient beds lined the walls of the dormitories. There was no separate lounge or day room for patients to escape from the monotony of the dormitory or the bizarre behavior of their fellow inhabitants. The stem of the T was a long corridor flanked by treatment rooms, offices, a conference room, and a nursing station that provided service for the patient area. The basic color throughout the whole building was a bilious green. The walls were dark green tiles up to shoulder height and, above that, painted green walls. The ceilings were the same shade of green. Black linoleum floors shined after nightly polishing. I was told that the darker colors were supposed to be calming and soothing. I actually read somewhere that pink, red, or orange walls in psychiatric hospitals tended to stimulate violent behavior.

The San Francisco General psychiatric units were very busy places. Many patients would come and go daily. After a brief period of evaluation or treatment, the majority went home—or to boarding houses, residence clubs, halfway houses or wherever our very busy, creative and amazingly capable social workers could place them. One particular worker, Miss Stenstrom, took great pleasure in finding "homes" for people who had no other place to go. She was like a super-efficient firm but kindly grandmother.

As a sign of our growing effectiveness in patient treatment, helped by the increasingly frequent use of new antipsychotic drugs, only a tiny fraction of our patients were now committed to Napa or Agnew State Hospitals, our Northern California equivalents to Manteno. The patient populations of the psychiatric units, usually discharged after a short hospital stay, were immediately replenished by the San Francisco General emergency room, the only place in the city willing to accept behaviorally disturbed patients. These agitated patients were most often brought to the hospital by the police, who were empowered to place them on psychiatric 'holds'. Each of the patients was searched carefully by the nursing staff for weapons or items of self harm. I recall several people brought to the ER who had razor blades taped to the bottoms of their feet, or plastic bags filled with pills that had been stashed in a rectum or vagina. Once they were carefully searched, they were then placed in hospital gowns, placed back in restraints if necessary, and locked in one of a number of seclusion rooms attached to the emergency room area. There they waited until a psychiatric resident evaluated their candidacy for admission. If the seclusion rooms were occupied, some of the less disturbed patients might sit in a large emergency room waiting area.

Patients whose behavior had led them to gain access to the ER seclusion rooms usually merited admission to one of the psychiatric service evaluation units. The criteria for admission had some flexibility. If a patient had made a suicide attempt, or suicide gesture, or seemed about to harm himself or herself, admission was almost automatic. If a patient had been assaultive or

seemed imminently threatening, he or she was guaranteed admission. Severely confused or even less confused patients were usually admitted. Significant bizarre
behavior was also a common criterion for admission.

Usually about ten to fifteen patients were admitted
over the course of a single night, although at times the
number might be even larger. For each patient the 'on
call' resident wrote a series of management and treatment orders. Some orders were modified the next day by
the resident in charge of the unit to which the patient had
been admitted. The evaluation unit psychiatric residents
triaged the patients the morning after admission. Triage
meant rapid decision making. Within a few minutes the
resident would decide whether or not patients were to
be held on the evaluation unit for further appraisal or for
very brief treatment. Others were transferred to the two
treatment units. Still others were sent elsewhere such as
to the medical service or to jail. Occasionally a patient
was discharged outright.

Because of the sheer pressure of numbers and the
limited number of beds, things moved very fast. Unlike
my medical school experience at the University where
painfully slow evaluation was the rule prior to the com-
mencement of treatment, here at SF General aggressive
treatment was begun even before the patient left the
emergency room. This approach helped patients avoid
the massive regression we had all too often observed at
the University when we had endlessly evaluated patients
without initiating early treatment. In amazing contrast,

early intensive treatment led to results that were dazzling. The improvement rate was very high, and the time needed for effective treatment relatively brief. The majority of patients improved quickly and were discharged to a less intensive level of care and support such as a half way house, board and care facility, residence club, or home with a referral for out-patient treatment. The possibility of commitment and the chute to the state hospitals was still there. But the number of patients traveling down that chute was significantly smaller than it had been only two or three years earlier.

Reinforced by the arrival of new antipsychotic drugs such as Trilafon, Stelazine, Prolixin, and Haldol apart from the now old standbys of electroconvulsive therapy (electric shock treatment renamed to sound less sadistic), insulin coma treatment, and even psychotherapy, the psychiatric residents treated patients aggressively and fearlessly.

Because there was always intense pressure on the residents to vacate beds to make room for the new arrivals waiting in the ER seclusion rooms across the street, premature discharge was common-place, just as it is now. It seemed that all a patient needed to do to get out of the hospital was to say that he or she was no longer suicidal, or that the hallucinatory voices were either softer or gone altogether.

The practice of premature discharge often led to poor follow-up care despite the valiant efforts of our social workers. Patients would commonly discard the one month supply of medication we gave them at the time of discharge. And they would tear up their appointment cards to visit the outpatient clinics. These were the many patients who had not improved to where they could acknowledge that anything had ever been wrong with them. They didn't believe that they needed follow-up help. Because they had been inadequately treated, and because they had no follow-up care, some committed suicide. Others decompensated, and in an agitated psychotic state were later brought back to the hospital for another round of treatment. This scenario came to be called the 'revolving door' system. After awhile the police, frustrated with the futility of their efforts, came to pick up only those patients whose behavior was most egregious or most dangerous.

Some of our patients were clearly violent. At his best, Dietrich looked like a glowering, tattooed muscular giant. At worst, when he walked down a major San Francisco street brandishing an iron pipe, even tolerant San Franciscans recognized that he was dangerous, and they scattered before him. He was shouting that he was going to "fight the Commie bastards" who, he claimed, were following him. He was apprehended by the police and brought to San Francisco General. After a few days on the men's evaluation unit he was discharged when he quietly explained that he "did not want to have anything to do with them Commies."

At the time of discharge the whole staff knew that Dietrich would not follow through with an after-care appointment, and that he would be readmitted within a few weeks. When, as predicted, he reappeared in the emergency room, the staff just said, "There's Dietrich again. He's a chronic." Hoping that nothing really bad would happen, we would try to overlook his dangerous potential and follow the same sequence for inadequate treatment and repeated admissions.

Dietrich was a good example of how a patient became a casualty of the revolving door system of hospital psychiatry. He never received a long-enough period of hospital treatment to prevent his regressing... again and again. Whatever potential he had to be free of psychosis was never realized. I believed even then, and still believe now, that the potential for being psychosis free is very real for the vast majority of patients. Yet by inadequate treatment we made Dietrich and the many like him into "chronics." If they came to the emergency room too often or became annoying to the staff, they might end up on the chute to the state hospital.

I was one of five residents on the San Francisco General Psychiatric service. We were the doctors who did all of the day to day work of admitting, treating, and discharging patients. Four of the five doctors came from the Langley Porter Neuropsychiatric Institute, a branch of the University of California medical complex in San Francisco. Their rotation at San Francisco General was for six months. My stay, as the sole representative of the Mount Zion Psychiatric Clinic, was to be for a whole year.

The Mount Zion Psychiatric Clinic unofficially overlapped with the San Francisco Psychoanalytic Institute.

The two institutions represented the two opposing camps, or schools of psychiatry, of the era. Langley Porter was the bastion of organic psychiatry. All mental illness, according to this school, stemmed from biological factors. Meanwhile the psychoanalysts back at Mount Zion believed that psychiatric problems stemmed from unresolved problems dating back to childhood. They viewed the organicists as unfeeling, uncaring sadists who delighted in giving patients electroconvulsive therapy, insulin coma, and lobotomy. According to the psychoanalysts, the organicists were now caught up in the newest dehumanizing approach of drugging people and turning them into mindless robots—a kind of chemical lobotomy.

The organicists had their own not-too-kind view of the psychoanalysts. They believed that the psychoanalysts never cured anyone and never got anything done. They perceived the psychoanalysts as a kind of fraudulent joke, well portrayed in the *Psychoanalysis* comic books available at the time. Their idea was that the psychoanalysts pretended to treat the 'worried well', while avoiding patients with real mental illness.

Not surprisingly, if a psychiatrist at this time in history claimed to be an eclectic, one who sought to use the best concepts and techniques of both schools of thought, he was regarded by both sides as basically ignorant. He was judged incapable of mastering and employing the vastly differing concepts and techniques of either major school.

The very existence at the time of 'schools of thought' indicates how primitive the field of psychiatry actually was. Rather than a healing science, schools of psychiatric thought were more like different religious faiths, each proclaiming its monopoly on truth. And I, with my intense belief in psychoanalysis was, at least up to then, a neophyte apostle of one of those faiths.

Dr. Gloria Bentinck and an assistant psychiatrist, clear-cut organicists, were in charge of the San Francisco General psychiatric service. Even before I arrived at San Francisco General, I had been forewarned that Bentinck barely tolerated having a Mount Zion resident on her service. I knew I would face a nonstop struggle to save patients from insulin coma, electroconvulsive treatments, and excessive drugging. I envisioned that once I had rescued them, I would have the opportunity to help them recover through psychoanalytically-based psychotherapeutic techniques.

At the time of my arrival, Jules Weiss was the Mount Zion resident who was just completing his first year of training. It was his place that I was taking. Jules was serious, energetic and very bright. He spoke rapidly with a polished voice. He had so much to say that he seemed compelled to talk fast. Everything he said underscored how much he had learned during his San Francisco General year. He seemed to me the living proof that I was on the right career track, and that the program I had chosen was as good as it could possibly be. Jules had already been accepted as a candidate for the San Francisco Psychoanalytic Institute. I could see that he was well on the way to becoming a psychoanalyst, and I was eager to follow in his footsteps.

My orientation day with Jules provided one surprise after another. I was amazed that he never once mentioned psychoanalysis or psychotherapy for treating serious mental illness. Instead he talked about the excellent results he had seen from the use of Thorazine, and even newer drugs like Trilafon and Stelazine. He talked about what these drugs were and how best to use them. He told me about involuntary movements that might appear as a side effect of the drugs, and medications like Artane or Cogentin that should be given to make the movements go away or to prevent them from occurring in the first place. Langley Porter residents, he noted, had been instructed to wait till the involuntary movements appeared before they administered what they saw as an antidote. Jules thought it inhumane to subject patients to the needless discomfort of involuntary movements when prevention was possible. He also advised me to prescribe high doses of the antipsychotic drugs for most patients in order to get the best results, doses significantly higher than those recommended by the pharmaceutical companies. He did warn that an extremely high dose of Thorazine, exceeding 2000 mg. per day, had induced an epileptic seizure in one of his patients. He had already observed that one new medication,

Compazine, seemed totally ineffective in treating psychotic patients even though it was chemically related to the other new and more effective antipsychotic drugs.

Jules then expounded on electroconvulsive therapy. What he described was much different and far more safe than the punitive and hazardous procedure I had seen at Manteno. Instead of the trauma of a series of mini-electrocutions, patients were now put to sleep by an intravenous anesthetic. They were then given a powerful muscle relaxant, succinyl choline, so that at the time of the electrical treatment a patient was so relaxed that the convulsion itself was barely noticeable as a minor muscle spasm or small jerks of the patient's feet. In addition, patients breathed oxygen before they were put to sleep. That way they did not use up inordinate amounts of oxygen in their bodies before they began to breathe normally again after the electrical treatment.

Prior to being given electroconvulsive treatment, prospective candidates all had X-rays of their necks, chests, and backs. Jules noted that this procedure enabled us to screen out patients whose preexisting back problems might be aggravated by the treatment. The screening and the treatment procedure itself sounded so much safer and more humane than the torture-like electrocutions I had witnessed at Manteno.

Jules explained that insulin coma treatment was also the responsibility of the residents. As he talked about insulin coma, his enthusiastic tone completely disappeared. His voice sounded as though he had been mechanically performing some distasteful task in which he was not actively involved. Jules then disclosed that while he was in charge of the insulin coma treatment program, one patient had died. From his facial expression I could see that he didn't really want to talk about it. But I insisted. Jules concurred with what I'd heard earlier, that the death rate from insulin coma treatment really was one to three per cent. Clearly when one of your own patients died, it no longer sounded like some text book statistic.

Patients were chosen for electroconvulsive treatment and insulin coma therapy from those admitted to the evaluation units. Dr. Bentinck and her associate usually chose the candidates for the treatments. Jules believed that Bentinck picked far too many patients for electroconvulsive or for insulin coma treatment; often these were patients, he thought, who could have been better treated by psychotherapy and medication.

As I listened to him, I naively hoped that during my tenure at San Francisco General I would be able to convince Bentinck that psychotherapy and medication would really help almost all of the patients now consigned for electroconvulsive or insulin coma treatment. And filled with the excitement of youthful optimism, I resolved to embark on a one-year crusade to save as many patients as possible from the dangers of these organic treatments.

Now I was ready to take on my role at the San Francisco General psychiatric service, whatever it might be. After what had seemed like a life time of waiting, at long last as a bona fide psychiatric resident I was to be given a hospital unit of my own. This wasn't to be like Manteno where no one had been discharged from my unit in years. This was a different kind of place, and at a different time in history. More treatment tools were at my disposal. I knew I could produce positive results. My patients were going to get well!

Apart from a ten minute talk with Dr. Bentinck, there was no orientation. I was assigned to a unit. The charge nurse, a crusty veteran of many years of service, gave me a rough idea of what I was supposed to do. But apart from the routine of the charge nurse there was no established formula for running a unit. The tradition had been for doctors to interview patients and to write orders regarding patient care. The orders were put into effect by a nursing staff which included the head nurse and a few registered nurses along with other less skilled personnel. Most of the time the staff did the best job that they could. They usually, though not always, used good common sense.

While I was to be working at San Francisco General Hospital, Mount Zion Clinic had assigned me two psychiatrists as supervisors. And each week I visited them at their offices to talk about anything that seemed to be my concern. Bob Towne heard all about my Manteno experience. After he had listened patiently to my description of what was going on at SF General, Towne said, "All you have there now are patients living in a big room. Why don't you make a real hospital out of that place?" He explained that my unit had no organization and no treatment program. The hospital unit could be and should be far more than merely a place inhabited by patients sitting around between daily psychotherapy sessions or other types of treatments. He recommended that I read Stanton and Schwartz, *The Psychiatric Hospital*, as well as Maxwell Jones, *The Therapeutic Community*. Over the next week I read the books he had suggested and, inspired by what I had read plus Towne's encouragement, I developed a plan for starting up a treatment program on my unit.

When I announced my plan for organizing the unit first to my charge nurse and then to the rest of the nursing staff, the idea of which now sounds so ordinary, simple, and straight forward, they thought it unique and innovative. I, as the attending psychiatrist, would conduct a staff meeting every morning to review the charts of all of the patients. As a treatment team, we were going to talk about each patient's progress or lack thereof. We were going to discuss diagnosis, treatment plans and changes in treatment plans related to the patient's progress. After the morning treatment staff meeting, we then were to have bedside rounds three mornings per week. During these rounds we all, as a group, went from bed to bed and talked to each patient. I initiated a series of regular patient group therapy meetings. Some were intended to help patients to talk to one another. Other meetings were to encourage patients to talk about their problems if they were able to do so. The staff had discussions or feedback sessions after each group therapy meeting. In addition, I tried to see most of the patients in individual therapy sessions.

When Bentinck heard about the new unit program, she was furious. She called me into her office and demanded an explanation. She was suspicious of what I was doing, and did not like the idea of my scheduling talks about patient care with the nursing staff. The staff were largely uneducated, she said, and were not to be encouraged to voice opinions about patient treatment.

I did my best to explain my plan and to reassure her that this was not some radical rebellion. There was not a half-baked psychoanalytic revolution taking place on her turf. She calmed down, but when I left her office, I knew that she hated the system I was putting into place. Despite her objections that I was keeping the nursing staff from doing their real jobs, I did it anyway.

I never kept statistics about whether patients treated on my unit got better more often or improved more quickly. I suspected that they did. One unanticipated consequence of the increased patient improvement rate was skyrocketing staff morale. As they became a treatment team, the staff became energized. Newly empowered, they did much more to help patients. I heard rumors that nursing staff from other units were requesting transfer to my unit. Only one nurse requested transfer off of my unit because this whole new way of treating patients upset her.

It was apparent that psychotherapy at San Francisco General was not going to follow the five basic rules I had learned in medical school and which had been so totally inappropriate at Manteno. Here at SF General, passivity by the psychiatrist was clearly contraindicated. I could not sit quietly and listen to a psychotic patient's word scramble. How could I sit in silence and listen while a patient recited the commands of nonstop auditory hallucinations? It was impossible to remain quiet when someone with suicidal despair made a cogent case for being dead to alleviate mental pain and anguish. And even for those patients who were coherent and whose grasp of reality was intact, there seemed to be little therapeutic value in silently waiting for them to divulge crucial information from which I as a therapist occasionally made meaningful connections. This was not Manteno or the University of Chicago. Some different approach was necessary to help patients get well. Patients here at SF General were expected to show demonstrable improvement almost day by day.

My second Mount Zion faculty supervisor, Joan Davidson, suggested I take an active role and talk to patients about what they were doing on the unit. For a psychoanalytically oriented doctor, this was almost a heretical concept. I was being advised not to talk to patients about their emotional problems. Davidson explained that when patients were overwhelmed by their problems, they were often in no condition to talk about them. She was advocating what ultimately became a central operational tenet in ego psychology. When a patient was overwhelmed, it was usually better to avoid talking about intense emotion laden problems. Then at some later date, when the patient had partially recovered, he or she might be better able to deal with what had been an overpowering issue.

Davidson suggested that I might even have patients write down what they did from day to day. Before long I had most of my patients writing mundane things such as what they had eaten at each meal, or how long they had slept, or whether they had showered. Each day I asked them to produce and review what they had written in their diaries. I urged them not to write down what was troubling them. They were to focus only on what they did. We then spent the therapy sessions reviewing what the patients had written. I often directed the patient's attention onto whether the writing was sufficiently detailed, and whether it made sense. I even focused on spelling and grammar. Based on my positive experiences with this technique, Davidson and I ultimately wrote a scientific paper, *The Use of Directed Writing in Psychotherapy*, which was published in a well-respected medical journal, *Bulletin of the Menninger Clinic*. I was proud of myself. Having a published scientific paper to my credit gave me the feeling that I was starting to make my contribution to a changing psychiatry.

Some patients prior to being admitted to my unit had become frightened and uncontrollable. Georgia was a 16-year-old American beauty with a pert nose, a long pony tail and a figure out of *Shape* magazine. Her mother reported that one night she had become confused, agitated and sleepless. She told her mother that she was scared. Then she began to run from room to room throughout the house. She became so agitated that her parents could not control her behavior. Fearful for her safety, they finally called the police, after which she was brought to the San Francisco General emergency room.

She was admitted to the evaluation unit, and the following day was transferred to the woman's treatment unit. When I first saw her, I was struck by her sweet and lovely face. But by then she had become a statue— mute, stiff, and incontinent, a classical case of catatonic schizophrenia. Since she was neither eating nor drinking, keeping her alive required that she be tube fed. The onset of her illness reminded me of the early stages of schizophrenia that Professor Nathan Apter, my mentor at Manteno, had described as the natural course of acute schizophrenia.

By now we were prescribing antipsychotic drugs to most psychotic patients, and Georgia was started on Stelazine. She was also given Cogentin to prevent the potential development of antipsychotic drug induced involuntary movements. Much to my disappointment, Georgia did not improve at all over the first week. She didn't talk. She didn't move. She refused to eat. And, because she refused to drink anything at all, we had to continue to give her fluids through the nasogastric tube.

To help Georgia improve, I decided to give another try to James Rosen's psychoanalytic approach to treating schizophrenia. When I had worked at Manteno, I had employed this set of new and radical techniques to treat patients whose serious schizophrenic illness had been of long standing. None of them had worked. At the time I had failed miserably to bring about any therapeutic change.

But this was a very different situation. Georgia's illness had only recently begun. Perhaps the Rosen techniques might be more effective with newly stricken psychotic patients. Rosen's treatment approach assumed that behind acute schizophrenia lay a basic problem between the patient and his or her mother that stemmed from infancy. My treatment plan was to intervene in the illness through a duplication of some of the patient's early life experiences and to provide her with what was then in psychoanalytic circles called a 'corrective emotional experience.'

I began to feed Georgia with a baby bottle while I told her again and again that this was healthy milk to make her feel good and to help her grow. "This is not the bad stuff your mother used to feed you." I told her repeatedly how she was safe, and that no one would abandon her. I knew that the approach seemed very bizarre in itself. Yet that was what was advocated in some of the respectable psychoanalytic literature of the day.

One day in the middle of a feeding Georgia suddenly grabbed the baby bottle from my hand and threw it against the wall, screaming out, "I'm not a baby!" I was startled. This outcry had been her first verbal utterance since admission to the hospital. It was then that I realized that patients with acute schizophrenia could not really be helped by attempts to gratify frustrated infantile needs. Maybe they did have unconscious problems with their mothers stemming back to infancy, but we couldn't help them with feeble attempts to recreate a positive infancy experience.

Suddenly free from the bonds of my previous framework of thinking, a whole new set of ideas for treating schizophrenia came pouring into my mind. We might be more helpful by directly assisting psychotic patients to strengthen their defective grasp of reality. We could enable them to firm up their vague, fuzzy, or rambling thinking. We could help reduce their catatonic stiffness and their problems with eating. We could fight against their withdrawal from the rest of the world. Patients could be aided in modulating their outbursts of intense emotion.

These were the kinds of problems that we—the treatment team surrounding our patients twenty-four hours a day—could actively address in Georgia's treatment. There were to be no more baby bottles. I ordered the staff to get Georgia out of bed and to keep her dressed in clean gowns or street clothing, even if she were to soil herself. I asked that she be taken to the dining tables for meals with other patients. She would need to be spoon fed if she did not eat by herself. She was to be assisted and encouraged to do as much as she could possibly do. As members of the treatment team we would all point out to her what was real and what wasn't real. We also tried to help her make sense when she talked, telling her when her speech sounded confused and jumbled. We helped her to move her stiffened limbs through passive movements by the staff, almost as though she were in physical therapy. We reminded her repeatedly that she was ill, that she was safe, and that we were going to help her to get better.

To our delight Georgia improved significantly over the next few weeks. She began to dress herself, to eat normally, to wash and shower, and to walk around the unit without prompting. She still seemed dazed. But she became more and more capable of normal speech. She never talked about problems in her life, even though I asked about them every day. She insisted that everything in her life was fine. By the time she was discharged a few weeks later, she acted and talked as though she had never been ill. She never could acknowledge the very existence of her illness. Georgia demonstrated the massive denial of illness we commonly see when patients have recovered from an acute psychotic episode. She wanted to forget about her illness the same way we all want to forget about last night's bad dream.

Two weeks after Georgia was discharged, to my amazement her mother was admitted to the psychiatric unit with almost the same symptoms. She too was catatonic. I was excited. What did it mean? It couldn't be a

coincidence. Somehow it had to do with Georgia's relationship with her mother. But what? I could only speculate. Did Georgia become psychotic as the price for
her becoming more independent of her mother? Did
her mother become ill as she felt Georgia was growing away from her? I never got to know the answer.
Georgia's mother recovered quickly, and both mother
and daughter dropped out of treatment.

Psychiatric patients often went away like that, seemingly just disappeared. While there were always plenty
of new patients to replace them, that didn't stop you
from wondering how some of the others had turned
out. Did they stay well? Or did they become sick again,
but not to the degree that they ended up back in the
hospital?

Leon, a middle-aged engineer, called the police and
the FBI to warn them that foreign agents were planning to
blow up the Panama Canal. Those days, anyway, such a
warning was a likely sign that someone had a serious personal problem, and over his vehement protests, Leo was
brought to San Francisco General for admission to one of
the psychiatric units. He was an unmarried, friendless man
who lived alone in a one-room apartment. His flabbiness
attested to his unfamiliarity with physical exercise. When
questioned, he denied that he had any sort of problem
except for the government's unwillingness to listen to him.
He had elaborate workbooks and blueprints of the canal
and what he saw as the sinister plot to destroy it.

At first I challenged his delusions about the canal. I told him that he had an illness and that his ideas about the imminent destruction of the canal were not real. But he had total conviction in his delusional system. No matter what I said or how often I said it, he ignored my comments. His response might be to calmly elaborate his delusional concerns in more detail in order to withstand the attack of my arguments. After a week I realized I could not successfully challenge Leon's fixed delusional system. His conviction in the plot to blow up the canal was lodged in mental concrete. I took to listening to the details of the plot. Our sessions became filled with his explaining the problem to me. I began to caution him against telling other people about the plot lest they think he were crazy. I advised him that government agencies really did not understand, and that to stay out of trouble (jail or the hospital), he needed to keep his concerns about the canal more secret. It seemed to work. He began to talk more about his job and minor problems with his peers that seemed major to him.

In my efforts to treat Leon I had rediscovered that it was almost impossible to successfully confront a fixed delusional system head on. After a month of treatment, Leon was discharged to live in his apartment and to return to work. I never saw Leon again. From time to time I would wonder about him. Later you couldn't help wondering, of course, how Leon's story might be received in post 9/11 years.

The telephone usually began to ring sometime around midnight. The message was always the same. "Dr. Widroe, we have someone here to see you" said the voice on the other end of the phone. The 'on call' psychiatric resident slept in a small room on the fifth floor of the psychiatry building. When summoned, we went over to the emergency room across the street to evaluate candidates for admission. Waiting for us in locked, minimally furnished rooms were those whose bizarre, violent or self-destructive behavior had necessitated police intervention. They had been harvested by the police from all over San Francisco. No other hospital wanted anything to do with them.

The residents rotated the on call ER coverage. Most of the other residents dreaded night calls. They grudgingly did their duty as commanded and then complained a lot the next day. They reminded me of my fellow students in medical school. For them having fun had a top priority. Work was considered a secondary yet mandatory intrusion. I remembered the days when I had felt that way. But then living at Manteno State Hospital for three months just a few years earlier had changed all that.

My new job helping to save people in the ER had become my "fun." Strange as it may seem, my response to night call was quite different from that of the other residents. Each time the phone rang, I would awaken with a sense of excitement, almost exhilaration. I would actually run across the street to the ER. In my mind I wondered what kind of case I was going to see when I got there. Would it be someone whose condition I had never seen before? Would I be able to figure it out and lay out the right orders to start a very sick patient on the road to recovery?

Much of the time I found myself dealing with patients who had some variation of the many kinds of schizophrenia I had seen so often during my days at Manteno. But here the onset of the crazy behavior usually was much more recent, and the patients far more agitated. Quite often it was some violent or destructive or threatening behavior that had led to police intervention. Often my initial interviews with these patients took place while they were in leather restraints for everyone's protection.

Those who had made serious suicide attempts were dealt with as medical emergencies and treated accordingly on the medical service. Once they had improved medically, they might be evaluated by one of the psychiatric residents and then transferred to one of the psychiatric units. I got to see some of these patients along with others who were threatening suicide or whose attempts had failed for any number of reasons. Sometimes they may have vomited an overdose of pills. Self inflicted cuts had been patched or sewn up. A friend or family member may have arrived home unexpectedly and interrupted the suicide attempt. Or the suicide candidate had phoned someone to say good-bye who in turn had summoned life saving authorities.

Alcoholics and drug abusers in various states of intoxication or withdrawal were plentiful. I hadn't seen many of them before.

Even now I recall my first encounter with a patient suffering from delirium tremens. A middle-aged, ill kept, sweating, red-faced man was seated in the ER waiting room lobby only because at the time all of the psychiatric evaluation seclusion rooms were filled. After I had seen all of the seclusion room patients, the ER nurse pointed him out to me. "You have one more to see." When I approached and introduced myself, he suddenly sprang to his feet and began stamping on imaginary crabs and roaches. "Don't you see it? There goes one! There goes one! Help me get them!" It was amazing.

In another ER encounter I was amused with the couple who showed up, each demanding that the other be admitted to the psychiatric unit because he or she was crazy.

All this on top of a parade of patients with an infinite variety of schizophrenic, manic-depressive or depressive illnesses helped me sharpen my interview skills. I began to feel increasingly confident. By June 1959, the end of my first year of psychiatric residency, I believed that I had seen everything. I thought nothing could surprise me anymore.

Of course I was wrong. LSD, PCP and other drug-related psychopathology all lay in my future. Nor had I seen elderly patients with different types of dementia. In addition I did not recognize my almost total inability to diagnose and to treat the typically less florid but still serious psychiatric problems seen in day-to-day psychiatric office practice such as anxiety disorders, apathetic depression, attention deficit disorders, and situational stress.

How things had changed within only a few years! With the help of antipsychotic medications, we now expected very sick patients to improve significantly or to even become symptom-free within a few weeks. And they usually did live up to our new level of expectation. My dreams of helping people—so frustrated before— were now coming true.

I had managed my electroconvulsive treatment month pretty well. I'd given the electrical treatments carefully using the procedure of preoxygenation, intravenous anesthesia, and medication induced muscle relaxation. How radically different this was from shock treatment at Manteno where there had been no anesthesia, where patients didn't breathe until they turned dark blue, where the only protection against treatment-produced fracture or back injury meant being kept down by a sheet held by four other patients, each awaiting his or her turn for a treatment. Now some three years later, using the modern approach, there had been no injuries or complications, and many of the patients who received the course of treatments improved significantly.

Nonetheless I remained convinced that the majority of the patients whom Bentinck assigned for electrical treatment could have been treated with medication and psychotherapy. I argued with Bentinck a number of times during the year about which patients should be candidates for electrical or insulin coma treatment. She was almost always suggesting one or the other, and I was almost always opposed. Sometimes I got my way. I then felt I had to work extra hard with those patients, since their recovery would be proof that I had been correct. But no matter how often I proved my point through the evidence of patient recovery, our argument continued with each round of newly admitted patients. Despite our many treatment successes using medication and psychotherapy and the effectiveness of our well organized treatment program on the units, I could not convince Bentinck that her convictions about electroconvulsive treatment and insulin coma therapy were wrong.

After ten months at San Francisco General the moment of truth had finally arrived. It was to be my scheduled month to run the insulin coma program. There had been no deaths that year due to insulin coma. But the one to three per cent overall mortality rates described in the psychiatric literature, along with the death that Jules Weiss had talked about, left me seriously concerned. Why should we jeopardize anyone's life when we now were getting such great results from the new antipsychotic drugs plus psychotherapy? I agonized about the issue for weeks. I reviewed the old and the new literature on insulin coma to see if I was incorrect, or whether the number of deaths had changed. I felt much more comfortable with electroconvulsive treatment since new improved techniques had made the procedure so much safer. But according to the scientific literature, the mortality rates from insulin coma therapy remained the same.

There was no question in my mind about the life threatening dangers of insulin coma. The real question was how could I get Bentinck to stop prescribing it? Two weeks before I was scheduled to take over the coma program I went to her office to make my case. I presented all of my carefully prepared and well documented arguments. Reminding her of the insulin coma death at SF General that had occurred the previous year, I concluded with a statement that I should not be expected to administer a form of dangerous treatment that threatened patients' lives. I even went so far as to say that I would not do it, and I urged her to discontinue the program.

She was not the slightest bit happy or reasonable, and her response floored me. She asked if I had considered finishing my residency elsewhere. And she advised that I carefully reconsider my position.

Suddenly my whole career in psychiatry was in significant danger. I was certain that if I were kicked out of the SF General program, Mount Zion would boot me out altogether. And after that serious a career blemish, what other respectable psychiatric residency program would ever accept me?

My tension and agitation reached a level unlike anything I could recall. That day I couldn't concentrate on my work. But no matter how anxious I was feeling, the feeling was nothing compared to the level of dread I experienced the following day when I received a call from Mount Zion summoning me to meet with Dr. Norman Reider. Reider was the head of the psychiatric clinic and the Director of the San Francisco Psychoanalytic Institute. While I did not actually become catatonic, I had a new appreciation for the term 'scared stiff'. My whole career was in serious danger.

Two days later, fearing for my professional life, I was pacing the corridor outside of Reider's office. After I waited several life times, he suddenly popped out of his office, put his arm around my shoulder and said, "Widroe, I got this letter about you from Gloria Bentinck." He paused, and I think I stopped breathing. When he finally continued, he said, "Don't give her such a hard time. Some people don't take it very well." He then walked away leaving me sweating and speechless in the corridor. I had to sit down to recover.

That was all he said. What did he mean? It had been like God talking in thunderous tones. He never scolded me. He never questioned me. He never threatened me. I felt strangely comforted. I was still one of his lambs. I was in his good graces. It seemed as though God was on my side. He had given me profound advice, a bit vague, but I knew the answer was there—someplace in his words. Now it was up to me to figure out what to do.

After a sleepless night, I had the answer. When I went to see Bentinck the next morning, I began by apologizing for being such a pain in the ass all year long. I then acknowledged that she was the director of the service. In addition I pledged that I would do whatever was expected of me to the best of my ability. She could look forward to my more pleasant and cooperative attitude. Of course I would administer the insulin coma treatments, and I would welcome her review of my performance and any suggestions she might make. Whatever guidelines and protocols were already in place commensurate with patient safety, I would follow to the letter.

Of course this did not sound like me at all. Here I was talking to Bentinck as though I had abandoned all of my concern for saving patient's lives. Overnight I seemed to have been transformed into a coward. I had apparently deserted all of my principles for the sake of my own professional survival. Or was I wisely deserting a battlefield where all had been lost in order to fight a battle on another day?

The answer was neither one. I still had every intention of saving patients' lives. But I had a new strategy for doing it. The evening before my meeting with Bentinck, I carefully studied the San Francisco General insulin coma protocols, the ones Bentinck herself had written. The protocols stated that on the first morning of treatment a patient was to be given a trial insulin injection of ten units of regular short acting insulin. I knew that such a low dosage couldn't endanger anyone. The dosage was then to be increased by ten or more units per day five days a week until a dosage was reached that would produce coma. But with the explicit rationale of maintaining patient safety, the protocol permitted the insulin increment to be limited to as little as ten units per day. Following the protocol exactly as written, I then saw to it that no patient ever received more than the ten unit per day minimal insulin increment. The result was that during my tenure of running the insulin coma program no patient ever went into coma. Bentinck reviewed my patient records. She could find nothing outside of her approved protocol. Now the patients were safe from the specter of insulin coma death.

To my surprise almost all of the patients who received subcoma doses of insulin seemed to improve anyway. Subcoma insulin also seemed to have some significant place in our growing armamentarium of psychiatric treatments, a fact I later found confirmed in the psychiatric literature.

The insulin coma therapy program at SF General was discontinued within the following year. Had my struggle to keep patients away from the dangers of insulin coma produced any real impact on the program?

The contract between Mount Zion and SF General for a psychiatric resident from Mount Zion to follow in my footsteps was terminated after my stay. Economic issues were cited as the cause of the contract termination. Maybe?

X. FREUD DOESN'T LIVE HERE ANYMORE

Mount Zion Psychiatric Clinic was housed in a small modern one-story beige stucco building located across the street from Mount Zion General Hospital in San Francisco. Coming in off the street, one immediately entered the waiting room area. A counter separated just enough secretarial space for three full time staff. Behind the work area was the Director's office. At the other end of a long corridor was a good sized conference room. The corridor itself was lined with about ten identical small windowless therapy rooms, each the office of a second or third year psychiatric resident.

All of the offices were sparsely furnished with identical desks, desk chairs, patients' chairs, and couches. Patients occasionally would ask if they were supposed to lie on the couch. I was almost too embarrassed to tell them that I did not yet have a couch license, and that the couches here at the clinic were not really used for patient treatment at all. The couches served only as an empty emblem which announced that the Mount Zion clinic and the San Francisco Psychoanalytic Institute were closely related. All of the faculty at Mount Zion were members or advanced candidates at the Institute. Almost all of the residents in the Mount Zion program aspired to become psychoanalysts and begged and maneuvered for acceptance as Institute candidates. Everyone regarded Mount Zion as the junior Psychoanalytic Institute.

The reality was that the couches in our offices were only used for naps by residents, many of whom held moonlighting second jobs. I worked in a Kaiser Hospital emergency room on Sunday nights. That meant being up all night trying to treat patients with all types of injury or illness. While I got to be quite skilled at sewing up lacerations, I spent much of every Monday fighting sleep. A cup of strong coffee was my constant companion. I recall a patient reproaching me for nodding off during what was to have been a therapy session. The couch in my office looked very inviting to me, but, successfully fighting against the urge to sleep, I used it only once in my two years at the clinic.

Since the faculty were all psychoanalysts or at least advanced psychoanalytic candidates, the brand of psychotherapy taught was psychoanalytic in character. The psychotherapeutic process focused on digging into the childhood origins of patients' problems. Any psychotherapy which emphasized that the therapist be kind, directive and supportive instead of exploratory was considered a failure by the residents themselves, their peers, and their supervisors. We all tried to act like young psychoanalysts even though we were not really sure of what it was that we were supposed to be doing. Each of us had two supervisors to whom we presented clinical cases. We were criticized for any deviation from free associative psychotherapeutic techniques, the hallmark of true psychoanalysis.

Now that I was working at the Clinic, I was only one block away from the offices of the Psychoanalytic Institute, the Mecca of psychoanalytic thinking. Everything depended on being permitted to advance that one block and to ultimately attend seminars at the Institute itself. I forced myself to set aside any techniques I had learned or developed during my year at SF General in favor of a wholehearted effort to learn more about exploratory psychotherapy.

The patients at the clinic were so different from any I had seen before. They did not hear strange voices or see weird nonexistent things. They were not actively suicidal or homicidal. Most of them seemed very normal. Many were young people adrift in San Francisco trying to find out who they were and how to survive. Some suffered longstanding low-grade depression or anxiety which seemed to be misshaping their lives. Still others were making a mess of their lives with repeated patterns of behavior showing quite poor judgment.

At Mount Zion we did not see many patients whose symptoms were of recent onset. Because the clinic was very popular, it had a long waiting list for appointments. Evaluations for treatment were typically scheduled months in advance. By the time we were able to see them, prospective patients who had been in crisis often had improved significantly. We used to joke that many acutely ill patients got well because of 'waiting list therapy.'

It took many weeks before I came to recognize and understand the psychiatric problems I was trying to treat. Our supervisors tried to teach us about the often unconscious forces that led to the development of psychiatric symptoms or maladaptive behavior. We then attempted to help our patients understand their unconscious conflicts so that they might make more conscious choices in determining their actions or attitudes. They might learn to become free of repeating the self-destructive patterns of behavior to which they had been driven by now unconscious conflicts stemming from early life.

As I had hoped for so many years, I was finally admitted as a candidate to the Psychoanalytic Institute. Part of the process for becoming an analyst was for each candidate to become a psychoanalytic patient of a designated training analyst. I would have to lie on the couch and free associate just like any other psychoanalytic patient. After the first year of a three to four year period of psychoanalysis, a candidate might then, if the training analyst approved, be permitted to begin seminars at the Psychoanalytic Institute offices.

I was never sure of why all candidates had to become patients or "analysands." I did not feel sick or especially troubled. My life seemed to be on track. I was married with a young son. I liked my work, and I felt I was being successful both as a student and as a clinician. At the time I supposed the training analysis had to do with each candidate learning what a patient undergoing psycho-analysis goes through by being in the patient's position. I wondered what distinguished a training analysis from regular therapeutic psychoanalysis. I never found out. I raised these questions with other candidates like Jules and Harry and David. No one was able to tell me what training analysis meant. Nonetheless they all seemed happy with the arrangement. They felt it was personally helpful for their comfort and growth.

At that time in history there was something revered about psychoanalysis that permeated the society. Once when I was speeding to an analytic session, I was pulled over by a police officer. When I explained that I was enroute to my analyst's office, the officer quickly dismissed me with barely a warning. Then as an after thought, he asked if I were late for my session. Even more remarkable, to be sure I got to my session on time, he provided me with a siren-blaring motorcycle escort to my analyst's office.

Regarding my own analysis, I didn't share the plea-sure of my fellow candidates. Whenever my first analyst, Emmy Sylvester, talked, it always felt as though she were scolding me. Her curly gray hair matched that of the two giant Poodles almost always present in her office. While lying on the couch during my analytic sessions, I frequently heard snoring noises or the sound of passing gas (which I presumed came from the dogs). Once one of the dogs jumped on top of me during a session. I protested, but I was secretly amused. For a brief moment the sacred chamber of the psychoanalytic session had become an ordinary room with two people, some furniture and a pair of friendly dogs.

After an initial period of excitement, I became less and less enamored with the whole procedure. Of course any criticism of the procedure, no matter how reasonable, was considered a 'resistance' in the analysis which had to be further explored. Four sessions a week at the analyst's office was time-consuming and inefficient. It was also very expensive. We candidates had to pay regular rates for our treatment. No health insurance covered the cost of psychoanalysis or any other kind of psychiatric treatment, and there were no training grants. Training analysts did not give discounts and did not extend credit. In response to my inquiry, Sylvester had said, "Why should I be your banker?" I had to borrow money from my father to be able to afford my analysis. Good old dad! He never questioned what the money was for once I explained that it was to advance my professional career.

If becoming a psychoanalytic patient was the path to get through to my goal of becoming a psychoanalyst, I was ready to do it, no matter what it took. I did learn a few things about myself during the process, but not very much for the time and the cost involved.

After a year I changed analysts in the hope that working with a different training analyst might be more productive. My second analyst, Stanley Goodman, was a much more pleasant person than Sylvester. Goodman talked more often. Far more important for me, his tone of voice was kind. That alone made me feel that he was allied with me in trying to achieve something. But even with Goodman I did not find being a psychoanalytic patient to be productive or rewarding.

I couldn't help comparing my experience as an analytic candidate "analysand" with my having been a psychiatric patient during my junior year of medical school. I had just been jilted by a girl friend, the first intense love of my life, and I was bereft. I then saw a psychiatrist, Dr Robert Brockman, who was very helpful. Brockman had been talkative. He asked questions, and he offered concrete suggestions, some of which I followed. Within a few weeks I felt much better, and my life went back to normal. Compared to my psychotherapy with Brockman, psychoanalysis seemed to be a very weak therapeutic tool, especially if I couldn't figure out what part of me was being treated.

Psychiatric medications were rarely used at the Mount Zion Psychiatric Clinic. There was no administrative edict that they not be prescribed. That they were not used was more a function of psychoanalytic tradition. Besides, no member of the faculty had any experience with the use of psychiatric medication. Through my year at San Francisco General, I already had more experience in using psychiatric drugs than any of the Mount Zion faculty.

Because of the clinic's extreme psychoanalytic focus, no one on the faculty or even most of my resident peers seemed willing to prescribe psychiatric medications. Nor did they want to listen when I described some of the positive effects of antipsychotic drugs I had witnessed. That I had seen incredible, almost miraculous, treatment success made no difference. They were so entrenched in the practice or the pursuit of psychoanalytic techniques that they were actively resistant even to the idea of anyone prescribing psychiatric drugs.

Many, but not all, of the very bright faculty members whose opinions I usually respected made very foolish comments about psychiatric drugs. After awhile I lost respect for them.

Their commonplace arguments were echoed in some of the respected psychiatric literature of the time. For years I heard and painfully, often heatedly, disputed the same arguments I'd seen repeated in different venues.

Most commonly I heard "They don't really work. They just sedate people." Again and again I heard these claims from clinicians who had almost no experience whatsoever with psychiatric medication. By contrast, I could cite case after case, totaling hundreds of patients I had successfully treated at San Francisco General. Most were not sedated at all. I was puzzled that such intelligent people could demonstrate such a massive denial of reality.

The faculty and even most of my peers also had no understanding and refused to see that there were huge differences between antipsychotic drugs and sedating tranquillizers. They asserted that with the use of antipsychotic drugs no one could stay awake to function. I argued that the medications did work, that tranquillizers and antipsychotic drugs should not be bundled into one class of medications. There were any of a number of non-sedating antipsychotic medications such as Prolixin, Stelazine, Proketazine or Haldol which enabled patients to be up and around and even to go to work and perform well.

A second argument I'd hear was that all we drug prescribers were doing was enabling patients to mask symptoms no longer available for psychoanalysis. This claim assumed that psychotic or depressive symptoms were the products of unconscious conflicts that could be totally cured by psychotherapy alone. I retorted that patients free of severe symptoms seemed much more capable of exploring serious problems in their lives, while patients overwhelmed and preoccupied by psychotic symptoms or intense feelings stood no chance of dealing with major life issues other than the symptoms themselves. They could only pay attention to how miserable they felt. The medications, I asserted, did not mask conflicts. They enabled patients to become sufficiently grounded in reality and comfortable enough to think and talk coherently about their problems.

Another argument I heard frequently was that the very act of prescribing the drugs contaminated the 'transference'. The term 'transference' referred to the way patients had come to feel about their therapists. If the therapists said almost nothing and did almost nothing, the transference feelings about the therapist presumably became a projection of the way the patients had felt about their parents early in life. Examining the transference then became an important part of a patient's psychotherapy.

The mere act of a doctor prescribing medication was considered so meaningful that it was presumed the relationship between psychiatrist and patient might come to focus on this transaction alone. Similarly, it was felt that other significant issues in the therapy might become neglected. Yet in my own experience I found that prescribing medication caused no adverse effect on my therapeutic alliance with my patients nor any bad effect on my efforts at psychotherapy.

I began to feel contempt for some of the psychiatrists who focused their objections to the use of medication on such foolish arguments. These psychiatrists and psychoanalysts had become so enamored with the practice of psychoanalysis that they had forgotten what we were supposed to be doing in the first place— that we were physicians trying to help patients to feel better and to lead better lives. With little interest in patient care, they seemed more concerned with protecting the purity of the psychoanalytic procedure.

Yet another argument against the use of medication was that patients would be made too comfortable
and then lose all motivation for solving their problems.
The patient and the drug would wander off on a symptom free honeymoon, after which the patient and his
pill bottle would then drop out of treatment. I strongly
argued that this rarely happened. Patients almost never
were made that comfortable from the medications we
prescribed for them. After all, we were not prescribing
heroin. We almost never prescribed barbiturates. From
experience, I could acknowledge that a large number
of patients who recovered from an acute psychotic episode denied that anything had ever been the matter
with them. But this phenomenon occurred whether antipsychotic drugs had been used or not. Massive denial
by patients that they had ever been ill was, of course,
often an unfortunate part of the process of healing from
a psychotic episode. Sadly, it was their denial that they
had been ill that led them to avoid follow-up treatment
and greatly increased the odds for a relapse. But this
had nothing to do with the use of psychiatric drugs.

It all seemed strange. Here I was at the Mecca of
psychoanalytic teaching. For years I had yearned to be
here. But based on my own experience I had a different body of knowledge about a great new therapeutic
tool than anyone around me. And no one around me
wanted to share that information. This new information
about psychiatric drug treatment was clearly perceived
as an intrusion and even a threat to a true belief system,

and it upset most of the true believers. I felt alone, yet also empowered.

Eventually, by 1961 many others in medicine outside of the Psychoanalytic Institute were starting to pay attention to the value of psychiatric drugs as a new dimension of treatment. Even though I was still a psychiatric resident, I was invited to give a lecture to the Mount Zion Hospital medical staff on the proper use of psychiatric drugs. I felt flattered. I was now a young doctor being asked to teach physicians of all disciplines who only a few years earlier had been my mentors and supervisors. I loved spreading information that resulted in improved patient treatment.

Standing at the podium, I was pleased that the auditorium was packed with doctors, all curious about the new discoveries in psychiatry. But I was disappointed not to see a single member of the psychiatric faculty or any of my fellow residents.

Some problems we treated at the clinic were very serious.

"I am so depressed that I wish I could die!," one thirty-five-year-old woman told me. "I can't get out of bed in the morning, and I don't want to move."

While Nancy was stylishly dressed, her precise grooming was spoiled by non-stop tears wearing rivulets through her heavy mascara. She had come to the clinic without an appointment. My job was to perform an emergency evaluation. There was no doubt that she was severely

depressed, but she did not meet the criteria for mandatory admission to the inpatient service at SF General.

Regretfully I explained that the outpatient clinic
schedule was full, adding that I would put her name on
the clinic waiting list. I felt bad that I had nothing to offer
her. Then I remembered seeing a bottle of a new drug,
an antidepressant called Tofranil, which had mysteri-
ously appeared in a supply closet at the clinic. I did not
know anything about it. I hurriedly read a few instructions
from the package insert, then gave her enough medication to last a month. After she left the clinic, I started
to wonder what would happen if she took an overdose
of those pills. What if she died? I started to kick myself for
not being more careful.

Six weeks later her name rose to the top of the waiting
list. When she answered the phone, I was greatly relieved
to find that she was still alive. I invited her to return to the
clinic to talk with me about treatment. Just seeing her
in the waiting room I was struck that she looked like a
different person. She was smiling and laughing. "I don't
need treatment now. I feel great," she said. "I took all of
those pills the way you told me to. And I feel great."

Soon we were discovering the potential of a whole
group of tricyclic antidepressants like the Tofranil I had
given Nancy. The tricyclic name came from the shape
of a structure common to the molecules of members
of this drug family. At the same time, we began using
another group of antidepressants called monoamine
oxidase inhibitors, all related to the antituberculosis

drugs I had first learned about at Manteno. It took a few years to appreciate that there could be serious hazards associated with the use of MAO inhibitors. Some patients who took them had sudden blood pressure elevation and might even suffer from a stroke as a result. Doctors became fearful of prescribing them for their patients, and their use nearly disappeared because of the medical community's concerns. After this it would take decades for some psychiatrists to muster the courage and master the skills to employ them at all.

Perhaps only God or special men of great authority can give profound and powerful messages to those fortunate enough to come near them. The messages with the most power are those that are most succinct. Look at the impact of the Ten Commandments!

Dr. Norman Reider as both head of the San Francisco Psychoanalytic Institute and the Mount Zion Psychiatric Clinic was certainly a man with that kind of authority. One of his great gifts was his ability to relate to anyone so that they felt important, too. You knew who he was and what he stood for. And when he talked to you, at that moment you felt very special. For that brief moment, you shared the edge of his elevated existence.

When my friend Josh Hoffs and I were touring the country as senior medical students trying to figure out where we were going to apply for internships and residency training, Reider sought us out in a crowded auditorium full of the Mount Zion Hospital Medical Staff. "I heard you fellows were here visiting. Is everyone making you comfortable ?" For anyone to try to make a medical student comfortable was a foreign concept to us. No one had made us the slightest bit comfortable during all of our years in medical school. And no one had been the slightest concerned about our comfort at any of four other training programs we visited. At each stop we had felt like peons begging for attention. Yet here was Reider who surely had better things to do with his time, taking time out to make us feel special and wanted.

And it had been Dr Reider who had saved my career at San Francisco General Hospital the preceding year by telling me, in a few well chosen words, how to deal with Dr. Bentinck.

Most of the psychiatric residents barely saw Reider at the clinic. It was definitely a major event when we received notes asking, actually commanding, us to meet him in the clinic conference room after hours that same day. We were all there on time, waiting for what we weren't sure.

Reider came straight to the point without raising his voice. He said he'd received complaints from patients and some of our supervisors that we spent too much time and effort trying to be psychoanalysts. He said that psychoanalysis was not appropriate for most patients, a pronouncement we had never heard before. And this business of treating very sick patients by exploring unconscious motives and feelings was for the birds. Nothing good could come of it, he told us, my ears burning at his every word. "You need to help patients cover up primitive ideas and feelings that are pouring, unchecked, out of the unconscious and ruining their lives, or even endangering themselves or other people," he insisted, and called this 'covering up' process "interpretation upwards," a term I had never encountered either from my supervisors or in my reading of the psychiatric literature.

To make his point, Reider proceeded to tell us about some of his own cases.

Mary, who lived with her mother, looked and seemed normal at first glance. She had held an office job for six years. But, Reider explained, she was really very crazy. In her first therapy session, she talked a lot about daily urges to kill her mother. She described night dreams and daydreams of her mother's face and throat spurting torrents of very red blood while jagged splinters of glass flew all over. Reider ascertained that Mary had no actual plans for killing her mother, and that she had no history of violence in any form.

Reider's 'interpretation upwards' was, "Your mother must be a very annoying person. What does she do to irritate you so much?" As Mary, in response to his questions, brought up a series of what seemed to be minor complaints, Reider excused them all as products of her mother's own insecurity and fears. To us he explained, "Mary needs to have less anger toward her mother. If she is less enraged, she will be a happier person. She might even repair her relationship with her mother." To me

Reider's words were a bolt of lightning. This was permission, even a mandate, to use techniques different from the chimney sweeping, exploratory therapy approach we had all tried so desperately to emulate. I understood Reider. He advised us not to follow slavishly a technique that didn't apply to everyone. It had been as though we were attempting to perform appendectomies on all patients who came to see us, no matter what was wrong with them. He had told us to act like doctors, and that we should strive to put sick and impaired people back together. To myself I coined the term 'psychosynthesis', the opposite of psychoanalysis. I was too embarrassed to say it out loud, but it comforted me.

Reider continued to make his case for flexibility in patient treatment. Many patients in his private practice were young people dealing with issues of independence and issues of intimacy. One very attractive young woman dressed seductively and conducted herself in a most provocative way. At the same time, she complained at length about how men treated her as though all they wanted was to sleep with her. As Reider explained it, when she then reached forward to place her hand on his arm, Reider told her, "If you keep that up, I'll try to fuck you, too."

We were all stunned. How could he say such a thing?

He explained. "When I said it, I knew she wouldn't believe me. And she did get the point I was trying to make about how sexually provocative she was."

Reider went on to report the case of a middle-aged husband and wife who had bitter complaints about one another. In Reider's office they were openly vituperative, screaming at each other. Reider then talked to each of them privately, saying that the other had a serious mental illness and that the additional stress of the fighting was going to lead that spouse to a "complete nervous breakdown." He then gave them specific instructions on how to treat one another with an ongoing awareness of the fragility of the other.

We laughed in part to relieve our own discomfort. How could he be so dishonest? "It worked pretty well" was his explanation. Follow up visits suggested that there was a new level of civility in the household.

A fifteen year old boy was doing poorly in school. He reluctantly revealed that he heard loud critical voices most of the time, even when no one was there. Because of the voices, he could not hear his teachers and could not concentrate to read. Reider suggested that they do homework together during the therapy sessions. The therapy appeared to focus on completing his schoolwork.

Three years later Reider saw the young man on the street, and they had warmly greeted one another. His former patient reported that he had finally graduated from high school and now had a job. Reider asked, "Do you still hear voices?" The boy answered, "Yes. But it is your voice telling me that I am a good person, and that I can do things".

We were touched. Reider again explained that you had to match the therapy with the needs of the patient. You could not force all patients to fit into one particular type of therapy.

After Reider's case conference, I felt exhilarated. I realized that I no longer had to pretend to be a junior psychoanalyst, and I was now free to use whatever I had learned at San Francisco General in order to treat patients effectively. I could pay more attention to some of the more recent psychoanalytic literature, including the writings of Heinz Hartman and David Rappaport along with Anna Freud. These authorities had come to see psychological problems and mental illness as ego defects instead of the frustration of basic biological drives. The new psychoanalytic thinking was to center on ego psychology instead of the old biological drive psychology. Chimney sweeping techniques for the treatment of every patient was now history. This new focus encouraged us to develop varying and flexible treatment plans, as Reider had suggested. Patients were to be evaluated for ego function defects, and treatment plans were to be aimed at strengthening those specific defects.

I was eager to try out what Reider had suggested. And I had just the patient for it.

At twenty six Sara saw her life as a black hole. She had come to San Francisco at eighteen, fleeing from an incestuous relationship with her step-father. When Sara had pleaded for help, her mother insisted nothing was

wrong except for her daughter's overactive imagination. Once in San Francisco, Sara had hope for a new
life. But nights singing in a North Beach night club typically ended in her sleeping with admirers who had often
provided her with an income supplement. It was all old
and stale now, and there seemed to be no next step.

Over a few months her exploratory therapy brought
up a myriad of grisly accounts of molestation, surrender,
and self reviling. But there was no relief. If anything, her
despair seemed worse. Death seemed increasingly inviting and inevitable. As I watched her condition worsen,
I'd felt helpless in my efforts at treating her. I could envision a phone call from the coroner's office asking me for
information about her condition prior to her death. There
would have been an implicit indictment that I hadn't
done enough to stop her from killing herself.

One day she reported that she had been helping one
of the other girls at the club to sing better. Inspired by
Reider, I asked her if voice lessons might help my strained
throat. As I had hoped, she offered to help me; and her
therapy sessions came to focus on my hoarse voice. She
taught me specific voice exercises. She even massaged
my throat. When the other residents complained at the
loud 'MAAA-MAYY-MEEE' sounds exploding from my
office, we changed venue to the parking lot in back of
the clinic.

After a few weeks she reported that she had come
to look forward to our lessons. Even more important, she
began to feel brighter. She commented that for the first

time she was doing something for a man other than sex. After awhile I encouraged her to market voice lessons, and even to become a voice teacher. She felt good enough to follow my advice. The direction and the quality of her life improved. I couldn't wait to present that case to Reider at a resident's case conference.

Upon completion of my third year of psychiatric residency, I went into private practice. One year later I resigned from the Psychoanalytic Institute. From the time I started there, the seminars at the Institute had seemed dull and boring. Their basic thrust was still the psychoanalytic drive psychology of old. It was still all chimney sweeping. Was that all it was? After years of trying to get this far, it was an incredible disappointment for me! But now I knew that the path for effectively treating patients lay in a different direction.

I began to think about writing a psychiatric textbook, Ego Psychology and Psychiatric Treatment Planning, a "How To" book for psychiatrists and therapists. Its function was to describe how we younger psychiatrists and therapists might help patients repair damaged egos. While it seemed an awfully ambitious project for a psychiatrist just out of residency training, its real purpose for me was to advance my own education. I felt I needed to make up for something I'd missed during my psychiatric training program, and actually wrote the book not because I knew so much, but because I knew so little.

Up to that time the ego psychology literature was largely theoretical, and practical applications were nowhere spelled out. If I could puzzle through how to make ego psychology workable in day-to-day patient treatment, I hoped to become a much more effective psychiatrist. At the same time, by writing a book about it I might help psychiatric residents and other young psychiatrists and therapists avoid the highly limiting and often confusing path of classical psychoanalytic thinking. In the book, in words that might be acceptable to a psychoanalytically biased clinician, I even made a stab at explaining how psychiatric drugs worked. Treatment was no longer merely the application of techniques to dig at repressed events and feelings. As Reider had pointed out, the 'chimney sweeping' of old was way too limited. Treatment could now focus on how to make people stronger so that they could cope with stress—with other people, with their own impulses, and with life in general.

XI. TO BE OR NOT TO BE

The shabby Victorian two story gray house on Telegraph Avenue in Berkeley had at one time been modestly remodeled to house a half dozen psycho-therapy offices. Since then, except for paper towels and toilet paper in the shared restroom and the minimal evidence of the cursory passage of a vacuum cleaner, there was not a hint of additional maintenance. The run down house blended in well with the other dingy houses and buildings near the University of California campus. The office I sublet on Monday mornings had a cozy but worn out character. Its principal tenant, Dr. Kammerer, kept the office very tidy, every pencil having its exact place. The room itself usually made me feel comfortable and relaxed.

This particular Monday morning I was not so comfort-able, and certainly not relaxed. Lucy and I sat very still. Her gun was pointed at my chest; and from four feet away, she couldn't miss. While I could see Lucy on the other side of the gun, her smiling face now looked fuzzy and distant. In sharp contrast, the gun seemed to be growing larger by the second.

Lucy was 23, single, pretty, and worked as a filing clerk. Always freshly scrubbed and tastefully dressed, she looked ready to go to church on Sunday, though she had come for treatment of her depression. She had no history of violent behavior—certainly not of shooting anyone. How had it come to this? During her first four therapy sessions she often talked of feeling so bad that she wished she were dead. She explained that she'd felt this despondent for a very long time, ever since she could remember. When she had complained of feeling bad, her cold, self-absorbed mother had taken little time to listen to her and had done nothing at all to remedy her misery. Her mother had always been critical, and nothing Lucy could do was ever good enough.

While I knew Lucy had thought about suicide, I did not think she was actively suicidal; and it had never occurred to me that she might kill anyone—especially me. Obviously I'd missed something very important, and the price of my blunder was about to be horrendous. I was a very young psychiatrist, having completed my residency training just a few months earlier. Now I was amazed at what was happening, not to mention terrified.

"Is that gun loaded?" I asked. What a foolish question! Looking back I can see that my question was a product of wishful thinking mixed with fear.

It was 7:35 a.m.. Lucy's therapy session had started at 7 a.m.. Usually at seven in the morning I am wide-awake, but perhaps not at my sharpest. Today at 7:34 Lucy had pulled the gun out of her purse, saying, "Look what I've got." At 7:34 and two seconds I felt as though I had been given a jolt of intravenous adrenaline. I experienced surges of panic, against a background of sur-realistic disbelief. This was a bad movie, or a Sam Spade novel I had once started to read, or perhaps just a bad dream. Then why the hell didn't the alarm clock go off and wake me up? This was the moment described by people who while drowning recall a thousand memo-ries. My own thoughts accelerated to at least a few hun-dred per millisecond.

Was this real? Why was it happening to me? I had heard that now and then other psychiatrists had been killed by their patients. What had my one-time colleagues done when they were threatened? I couldn't possibly know. The other psychiatrists in my situation hadn't lived to describe what happened.

I felt very sorry for myself. I had just started my private practice—after all those years of training. I was married and had a two-year-old son. The promise of the life that lay before me was about to be turned off like a light switch.

What would Humphrey Bogart have done? Or John Wayne? James Bond would have thought of something to get out of this. Did Sigmund Freud ever have such a bad day? There was nothing I could recall in Freud's writings about how to handle this scenario. I bet no one had ever pulled a loaded gun on Freud.

I tried very hard to remember any lesson I had ever had during my psychiatric residency training, 'What do you do or say when a patient has a loaded gun pointed at your chest?' If there had been such a lesson, which I doubted, I must have been asleep in class that day.

In medical school one of my psychiatry professors, Dr. Nathan Apter, had a reputation as a hero for having single-handedly disarmed a gunman at one of the University Clinics. But I had never heard an account of how he had done it. During my psychiatric residency a faculty member had lectured us about death row murderers he'd evaluated—how many of them had had abnormal brain wave tests. A lot of good that did me now! Could I ask Lucy to put the gun away while I arranged for her to have a brain wave test?

With a tense, fixed, smile Lucy answered my foolish question, the one about the gun being loaded. "Of course it's not loaded." Half of me believed her because I so much wanted it to be true—that this display of an empty gun, maybe even a toy gun, was a symbol of how desperate she felt, a feeling she could not convey in words alone. The other half of me knew she was lying through her teeth. The gun was very real and very loaded. And something big-time needed to be done. I regretted never taking that martial arts class I had once read about. I had a flash image of kicking the gun out of Lucy's hand, just like in the movies.

I tried to read my watch without looking too obvious. It was now 7:38. Did I expect help to arrive at any minute? At that hour? What nonsense! Lucy and I were probably the only people in the whole building. I wished Dr. Kammerer would walk in and save me. It was really his office. While I sublet the office on Monday mornings, he was working at the University of California student health clinic. I could see Kammerer arriving at noon to find my dead body sprawled on his office floor. He would call the police who, I was sure, would soon apprehend my killer. What comfort that thought gave me vanished in an instant.

My frantic mind then shifted to magical thinking—where thoughts or gestures exert a supernatural control over reality—like knocking on wood makes a good thing happen. For me the magical thinking went like this. This isn't really my office. Therefore Lucy isn't really my patient. Therefore we should just stop pretending to be patient and psychiatrist and both of us go home. While I knew the thoughts were absurd, I was grasping for help from any place. I dismissed the whole notion and snapped back to my reality—the reality of Lucy on the other side of the loaded gun.

I now needed very much to be like Josh Hoffs, my best friend in medical school, who, like me, had become a psychiatrist. I admired Josh. He could think and act quickly. He always spoke clearly—with authority and good judgment. Once, at a cocktail party, his well intended hostess had pushed him into a room where he was faced by an agitated, menacing stranger. On leaving them sequestered, their hostess merrily announced, "George, this is Dr. Josh Hoffs, a great psychiatrist. He'll fix you." Josh saw that the man was terrified and very disturbed. He immediately said, "Look, George, I don't know you, and you don't know me. Our hostess is a kind person who means well and is trying to do a good thing. But tonight she made a mistake. I'm just another guest here at the party—just as you are. Why don't we go back to the others?" They had returned to the crowd in the next room, and nothing bad had happened.

So where was Josh when I needed him? This morning it was my turn to think crisply and to say just the right thing.

"Our time for today is up, Lucy. And we have to stop." Even when I said it, I knew it sounded stupid. Was that the best I could come up with? But I couldn't think of anything else to say. Josh would never have said anything that sounded so dumb. Yet I was so desperate to have this bad dream be over that I would have said just about anything. I then returned to reality and went on talking in a somewhat more sensible way.

" I think you are suffering a lot .You need to be in a hospital. I want you to put down the gun and go directly over to the hospital. I'll call over there and make arrangements for you to be admitted."

Silence. Nothing happened. About twenty hours passed at glacial speed all in the next sixty seconds as we stared at one another. I decided to try something else, the kind of stuff that in the hands of really good psychiatrists was supposed to lead to dramatic results.

"Look, Lucy, I'm not your mother. I'm not the cause of your pain and suffering. I'm your psychiatrist. And I am trying to help you. Why don't you put down the gun, and we can talk more about your going to the hospital so that you can be safe until you feel better."

Another forever moment of silence. Then we both stood up. I guess Lucy started to stand up first, and my move was almost a reflex. Both of her hands were now on the gun. Whatever denial I had had about the reality of the gun all disappeared. I now was certain that the gun was no toy, and that it was loaded. I felt helpless, weak, and sick to my stomach. There wasn't going to be a heroic move in which I diverted her attention and deftly kicked the gun out of her hand. I realized I was about to join the cluster of psychiatrists who had been killed by their patients. I tensed up to better withstand the pain I was going to feel in my chest—any second now. I could see that Lucy's arms were shaking.

There was an enormous explosion. And my ears began to ring. But there was no pain in my chest—or anywhere else. Only the bad smell of sulfur and a cloud of smoke. I was surprised. I was still alive, still standing. It was Lucy who crumpled to the floor. At the last instant she had turned the gun around and shot herself in the stomach.

For a minute I thought she was dead. But I wasn't sure. To ensure my safety, I kicked the gun away from her hand. I then knelt down to see if she were still alive. Her pulse was rapid, and she was cold and sweaty.

I grabbed the phone and hollered at the operator that I needed the police. It was a cumbersome version of calling for help in the pre 911 era. An odd thing then happened to me. Suddenly it was like the threat to my life had never happened. Lucy was the patient, and I was the doctor, trying to appraise her status and to be kind and comforting, telling her to keep her head down and not to move. I even reassured her that help was on the way.

How the paramedics and police arrived so quickly I don't know. But they did, and Lucy was whisked off to the hospital in no time. I recounted what had happened to a police officer who wrote down almost everything I said on a small tablet. Then he was gone, and I was alone—well, almost alone. The ringing in my ears was still there. But much more disconcerting was the visual replay of the experience with Lucy that started playing before my eyes—each time ending with a big bang. The bang, very loud, startled me each time the gun went off. The scene kept playing again and again, a video clip with Bose amplified Surround Sound, half in my head yet seeming totally real.

I phoned Dr. Kammerer, told him as best I could what had happened, and apologized for messing up his office. He didn't seem the least bit upset with me. He was always matter of fact and reserved. He said he would come to the office a little early to clean up further, and asked if there were blood spots on the Persian rug. I didn't remember if there were blood spots on his damn carpet. I was thoroughly annoyed that he didn't ask how I was feeling. I might have been the dead body messing up his Persian rug, waiting for him to walk in.

I drove around Berkeley for the rest of the morning, enjoying the sunlight, the run-down buildings, and the seedy looking students or street people in the neighborhood near the University. Still alive! STILL ALIVE!!! It was almost a loudspeaker blaring from my car as I drove along Telegraph Avenue. I coddled every image, noise and smell as though it were a precious jewel. My euphoric celebration of my own life and my enhanced sensations were interrupted every few minutes by the same involuntary video clips—always ending with a big bang. I had no control over it. I must have lived through the scene and heard the explosion of the gun hundreds of times. The interval between performances was sometimes only a few seconds. Then the next show began.

It felt very crazy. Fortunately I knew what it was. It's called traumatic neurosis; I had read several books about it during my residency. During World War I it was called shell shock. The WW I victims of shell shock were hospitalized, often for months, and then sent home, usually barely improved if at all. Many never got any better; and their lives were ruined with persisting symptoms of nightmares, flashbacks, extreme sensitivity to loud noises, irritability, weakness, depression, and fears about doing much of anything. They became emotional cripples.

During World War II Dr. Roy Grinker, while serving in the US Army in Africa, renamed the phenomenon. Shell shock became battle fatigue. To avoid the same out-come for his patients as the WW I victims, Grinker developed a radically different treatment approach. After twenty-four to forty-eight hours of observation at a field hospital a few miles from the battlefront, his patients were ordered back to active duty—often in the face of their vociferous protests. Back to active duty they went, and the vast majority fared well.

Following Grinker's advice I ordered myself back to active duty as a psychiatrist, and headed off to San Francisco where I had my own office. I had a handful of patients scheduled for that afternoon.

As I drove over the Bay Bridge toward San Francisco, I loved the sunny vistas, which now seemed extra bright and exquisitely beautiful. Monet and Renoir must have seen things this way. What would their paintings have looked like had they lived in California?

During my non-video clip and big bang moments, my mind focused on why the preponderance of people who ended their lives by jumping from bridges preferred the Golden Gate Bridge to the other four Bay Area bridges. While the other bridges were often more acces-sible to them, many even drove over the other bridges enroute to the Golden Gate. Something romantic about the Golden Gate Bridge invited tourists and suicide candidates. The other bridges all seemed so business like, almost forbidding people with suicidal intent from getting out of their cars to hurl themselves into the space above the Bay. It was as though the other busy drivers, racing to and from San Francisco, wouldn't let the suicide candidates stop their cars.

There was ongoing controversy about a plan to build a suicide barrier on the Golden Gate Bridge. It would serve to delay prospective jumpers, but might distract from the gorgeous views. One fool of a psychiatrist, whom I had known during my residency, opposed the barriers. A self proclaimed suicide expert, he argued that suicidal patients would find other ways to kill themselves if the Golden Gate were less accessible. Perhaps he was right to some extent, but jumping from the Golden Gate Bridge was deadly efficient. Survivors were rare—usually to the surprise of everyone, especially the patient. Other means of suicide, except for a gunshot in the mouth, seemed to yield a far higher percentage of survivors. Most depression victims, those who tried other ways to kill themselves, got another chance to live and to repair their lives.

As I drove to my office, life in San Francisco seemed very normal. The video plus the explosion kept playing in my head. No one in my office parking lot, the elevator or in my waiting room could see or hear the things I did. My patients arrived on time, and, for the most part, talked about the same problems they had had when I last saw them. Today I was the only one who was different. When I could, I tried to listen carefully and follow the treatment plans I had devised. I kept struggling against the urge to tell each patient who came into my office, "Guess what happened to me this morning. And I am alive to tell you the whole story!" But I didn't.

On the way home, the video continued. But by now the images were less vivid, and, with a great deal of effort, I could consciously insert a few changes in the script. In one version Lucy put down the gun. In another I took the gun away from her and emptied the chamber of its bullets. In a third the gun was really a toy gun, and we both laughed, but Lucy still went to the hospital. I couldn't stop the explosion from repeating—even in scenarios where Lucy didn't pull the trigger.

From my reading I knew that the nightmares would come. As predicted, they were there with their entire phantasmagoria. A lot of blood, searing pain in my chest, panic, my crumbling to the floor, my being pronounced dead by the police. I awoke sweating a number of times.

By the next morning, my mind was more my own. The intensity of the video clip, the loudness of the gun, the frequency of it all was lessened. Even the ringing in my ears was softer. A newspaper article based on the police report described what had happened. When I read it, it felt like they were writing about someone else.

A brilliant surgeon who labored many hours in the operating room had barely saved Lucy's life. Needless to say, Lucy had a new psychiatrist. I visited her once while she was in the hospital. We didn't talk about what had happened. It was all a painful fact of the past.

Perhaps there wasn't much to be said without some kind of emotional outburst by either of us. Lucy still wanted to be dead, and was subsequently committed to a state mental hospital. I never heard anything else about her.

For me, even when the dreams stopped, the ringing disappeared, and the video clip and gun shot noise were no longer frequent and involuntary, I was plagued with thinking about what had happened. The persisting question was what had I done wrong. What should I have done to prevent the disaster that had occurred? I called one of my old residency program supervisors to ask him to review the case with me. We went over it together in detail—a kind of therapeutic debriefing. It helped me feel better and regain my perspective.

I concluded that maybe there was nothing I could have done that would have prevented or altered the traumatic scene with Lucy. But I resolved that in the future I would try to be more sensitive to the pain and anguish of my patients, and to work much harder to give them relief.

XII. CRAZINESS AT U.C.BERKELEY

When I moved to Berkeley in 1958, it was a pleasant college town. By the time I left Berkeley thirteen years later, events had unfolded which made it seem that the world was turning upside down. This was to be the era of the Free Speech Movement, the Sexual Revolution, antiwar protests, and often pointless riots and destruction inspired, at least initially, by a small number of vocal student, non-student, faculty and community leaders.

Contrary to popular opinion, the number of protestors really was small. On any given day the number could be inflated by a group of students skillfully recruited between classes for a few hours of protesting or even rioting, especially if TV cameramen were about. The publicity was big, acting as a magnet to attract some anti-everything enthusiasts from all over. But the vast majority of us who lived in Berkeley were paralyzed spectators who wanted it all to go away so that we could do our work and take care of our families.

We Berkeley citizens were naïve, liberal idealists who regularly elected inept city council members who thought they could change the world—often at the expense of the community that had put them in office. There was always an "enemy of the people." After the council had designated the enemy as 'cars', we found ourselves dodging through an inane maze of concrete anti-car street barriers. When the enemy was identified as the 'capitalist utility companies', our council proposed moronic bills and initiatives to bring about municipal ownership of our utilities that would have resulted in our having dinner by candle-light.

The council, which, at best, was ill-equipped to go about the normal business of governing a small city, was totally befuddled by the lawless events on its streets. Their initial solution to illegal behavior was to make it all legal. For example, riotous demonstrations were supposed to become spirited community street dances. The council reasoned that if everyone could just have a good time and be happier, there would be no street violence. It was a bizarre policy of appeasement which in turn led to more lawless and disruptive behavior. Finally the National Guard was called in by then Governor Reagan to help restore order. When that ultimately happened, most of us were glad—although saddened by what had become of our community.

Having completed my psychiatric residency in 1961, I was no longer an "almost something." Now when I said I was a psychiatrist, it really meant that I was a psychiatrist. I felt as though I had finally arrived.

And of course I went into private practice. At that time almost everyone who was serious about a career in psychiatry went into private practice. Jobs in government clinics were always available yet served only as way stations for psychiatrists passing through to something else—often somewhere else. For a psychiatrist to have worked in a psychiatric clinic for more than a few years was to acknowledge poor training, laziness, or an unpleasant personality. While most clinic jobs offered tolerable pay, the parameters for patient treatment were never compatible with optimal patient care. And all psychiatrists knew it.

To some it did not matter. A steady paycheck with regular hours, infrequent night and weekend call, if any, set treatment protocols, and, not least, no ultimate individual physician responsibility did attract some psychiatrists—especially those who for lack of skill or personality problems of their own could never have survived in private practice. But to those new psychiatrists with energy, ambition, and flexibility and who strove to remain at the forefront of the field, the constraints of a clinic job were viewed as the institutionalization of mediocrity.

In contrast private practice has a special kind of allure. Individual private practice meant you were your own boss. You made the best clinical decisions you could. You bore the responsibility for those decisions. You got the 3 a.m. phone calls, and it was up to you to fix whatever problem came up. You worked as hard as you wanted to—often as hard as you could.

With much difficulty, you also made the business decisions. You determined your fees, your schedule, your charges, and you struggled with your costs. Young psychiatrists were then, just as they are still, poorly prepared for the business side of private practice. There had been no business management classes during medical school or residency training. Needless to say, we made one business blunder after another as we fumbled along. We didn't know anything about billing and collection. Nonetheless, it was now all up to us. It had become my responsibility to earn the income for my family. And despite much confusion and uncertainty about how to make it all happen, it felt wonderfully exciting.

In 1961 private practice in psychiatry meant solo practice. Psychiatric group practice was almost nonexistent, except in Southern California. From afar, group practice was viewed as somehow too mercenary and too restrictive to permit good medical practice. But no one really knew much if anything about group practice, and no one really cared. Group practice seemed a needlessly complicated way of doing business. There appeared to be no real need in psychiatric practice for the staff that comprised the infrastructure of a group.

Health insurance with mental health coverage was in its infancy. For health insurance companies to be more willing to provide any mental health coverage for plan members, better and faster outcomes were required. Psychiatric care had to be cheap enough for insurance carriers to be willing to offer it as a health plan benefit.

The increasing use and demonstrated effectiveness of psychiatric drugs was just starting to have a major impact. More antipsychotic drugs were available. Whole families of antidepressant drugs, including tricyclic anti-depressants and monoamine oxidase inhibitors (MAOI), were being used effectively by most all physicians with excellent results. New benzodiazepine tranquilizers such as Librium and Valium enabled people to function better with less threat of addiction than the barbiturates of the previous decades. Over time some of these drugs would be overused and create new problems, such as amnesia from the tranquillizer Serax. Meanwhile the improvement for many with serious problems was clear and dramatic. New data led to better and faster treatment outcomes. Psychiatric treatment was no longer apparently interminable. Better outcomes led to the possibility of psychiatric care health coverage as part of overall health insurance. Mental health insurance coverage at least for outpatient psychiatric treatment had now become affordable.

Psychiatric hospital insurance coverage was initially limited to acute care psychiatric units in general hospitals, since these patients had the shortest, thus least costly, average length of hospital stay. Little if any coverage was available at freestanding specialty psychiatric hospitals, where the average stay was much longer and consequently more expensive. And all coverage at state mental hospitals was excluded, since the duration of a patient's stay there was still judged to be interminable and the cost of care astronomical.

In outpatient practice, patients generally paid for their own psychiatric care. It was common for a psychiatrist to hand each patient a bill at the end of the month. Because this seemed a simple procedure, most psychiatrists did not have office staff. But others realized that the absence of support staff brought no cost savings at all. Professional time spent typing out bills and doing books was time very inefficiently spent. In comparison psychiatrists made the best use of their time by seeing patients.

There were already way too many psychiatrists in practice in San Francisco. Yet because I had trained at Mount Zion and knew many doctors on the Mount Zion Hospital medical staff, I hoped they would provide a network for referring patients if I dared to open my practice there. Having rented an office in a suite leased by a group of other psychiatrists, I bought my own furniture. I had no money to buy a symbolic couch, even though at the time I still planned to become a psychoanalyst. I envisioned that the couch would come later, when it really meant something. For now a few modern chairs and a desk would have to suffice. I then appealed to some of the medical doctors I had known to please send me a few patients. And they did! I was so thrilled when my first anxious patient came into the office. During that first session in my own practice I could barely tell whether I or the patient was the more anxious. The patient did improve with psychotherapy along with the use of a mild tranquilizer, Miltown. I was overjoyed when the referring physician called to tell me how much the patient had improved, and that he planned to send me more patients. What a nice guy!

Nonetheless, while I did get some patient referrals during my first six months of private practice, the total flow was just a trickle; an insufficient number to yield an adequate income. To make ends meet I continued to work as an emergency room physician one night a week, just as I had over the previous three years of my residency. I realized I would have to get a part time psychiatric clinic job to supplement my meager private practice income.

I'd heard about a large highly regarded student mental health clinic at Cowell Memorial Hospital on the University of California Berkeley campus. It was manned by many of the very best psychiatrists and psychoanalysts in the area. The twenty-seven thousand University students had easy access to excellent mental health care. To work at the Cowell Hospital psychiatric clinic was almost a privilege. The pay was low, but the professional atmosphere in the case conferences and even in the corridor discussions was reputed to be exhilarating.

Saxton Pope, a psychoanalyst, headed the psychiatric service. He was a thin, soft spoken, kind person who projected a regal image. He waved his cigarette the way a monarch might wave his coronet. Everyone he encountered regarded him as a benign prince. I candidly explained that I was looking for some part time work while I established a private practice. Pope said that he had no need for any additional out patient clinicians, but interjected that some very disturbed students might require up to thirty days of inpatient psychiatric care at the hospital. Would I have any interest in inpatient work? I jumped at the chance. I replied that inpatient work was my strong suit, that I'd had lots of inpatient experience. This was true, though I'd have said anything to work there.

Pope elaborated that Cowell Hospital had no psychiatric unit as such. Psychiatric patients were housed on the same floor as the medical and surgical patients. I had never heard of such a thing. Nor could I even imagine it. I envisioned a post appendectomy patient awakening from anesthesia to find a giggling schizophrenic standing over his bed adjusting the flow of intravenous fluids. How could such a system work without courting disaster? Yet I figured that it must work. They had been operating this way for years. As a veteran skilled in concealing my ignorance, I nodded my head in agreement. I hoped to indicate that the system made perfect sense to me, and that there would be no problem if I were hired. I must have appeared convincing. Pope hired me on the spot.

Four part time psychiatrists worked on the psychiatric inpatient service, with each of us caring for a handful of inpatients. We took turns being on call at any time of the day or night. A 'call' usually meant a trip to the emergency room to evaluate and take care of a student in crisis.

Cowell was a 120-bed acute care medical and surgical hospital located right on the University campus. Though psychiatric patients were usually assigned rooms along one particular corridor, the adjacent room often did house medical or surgical patients. On any given day most rooms could be used for either psychiatric or medical patients. Some of the rooms could be converted into maximal security rooms with locked doors.

There were no psychiatric nurses on the Cowell staff. Psychiatric patients were cared for by the regular nursing staff. A nurse might be assigned both medical and psychiatric patients. Cowell had only one male orderly in regular attendance, though an additional orderly might be called in to help with a violent or highly suicidal patient. University police could be summoned as additional backup.

Both the University police and the City of Berkeley police routinely brought severely disturbed students to the hospital for evaluation and admission or helped to return hospitalized psychiatric patients who had wandered away from the hospital and campus. While we could not rely on our limited manpower at the hospital to manage some of the acutely agitated patients, the system seemed to work. Less than one student per year required a transfer to hospitals with higher security units.

Each year seventy-five to one-hundred-twenty students were admitted to the inpatient psychiatric service. The average length of a student's hospital stay was nine days. After discharge, the patients were usually followed along as outpatients by the psychiatrist who had treated them in the hospital or followed by a therapist who had seen them prior to the hospitalization. What was amazing was that the vast majority of psychiatric patients who had been sick enough to require hospitalization were able to return to school and complete the semester.

I quickly learned how the system worked. When disturbed patients walked in or were brought to the emergency room by friends or police, the 'on call' psychiatrist would evaluate the patient and initiate treatment. When necessary we would attempt to sedate patients in the emergency room prior to their being admitted to the floors upstairs. The police would stay with us as long as needed. Once patients were manageable, they would be taken upstairs to hospital rooms by the nursing staff along with the police. A particularly disturbed patient might be put into leather restraints attached to his bed. If necessary, the door to the patient's room could be locked for everyone's safety.

The most common candidate for admission to the psychiatric service was a college freshman. The transition from the relative limits and comfort of home and high school to a raucous dormitory—plus an increased level of academic demand and the electrifying atmosphere of freedom without limits—simply overloaded many immature brain circuits. Unbridled intense feelings could all be amplified or distorted by drug, alcohol, and sexual experimentation. Guilt, anger, anxiety and poor performance often led to depression and a suicide attempt or an acute psychotic episode. Homesickness as such was rarely the problem.

I dreaded the morning phone calls I had to make to inform a mother that her nineteen-year-old daughter had been admitted to the inpatient psychiatric service the night before after an overdose of pills. There would be an almost palpable shock at the other end of the line. I would then hasten to reassure the stunned parent that their daughter was physically all right, and that she was in a protected environment. I'd tell the parents that I would have the patient call them within the next few hours. And, of course, we wanted the family to visit as soon as possible. I would offer to meet with them immediately after their arrival to help figure out the best course of action. After the reflex protective parental response of wanting to take their troubled child home, the most common plan was for the patient to continue in school and in treatment under the care of one of the clinic psychiatrists.

The hospitalized patients were seen by psychiatrists seven days a week. Each day the treating psychiatrist reviewed the patient's medical record, which included the nursing staff's up-to-date progress notes. The psychiatrist then talked with the patient and wrote his own progress notes and new doctor's orders. Finally he met with the nurse assigned to provide the patient's care for a discussion and update of the patient's treatment plan.

As the patient settled down, restraints, if they had been used, were removed. The door to the patient's room might be left unlocked, if it were judged that the patient no longer posed a threat to himself or to others, and that he or she was unlikely to wander off and get in trouble. With the permission of the doctor, the patient might begin to spend time in a TV lounge at the end of the corridor where he or she might be joined by ambulatory medical and surgical patients. With further improvement, psychiatric patients might be permitted to take brief walks out of the hospital or even to attend class provided they returned straight away to the hospital. Further improvement merited longer passes from the hospital, until the patient was finally discharged.

The University administration was very cooperative with what we were doing. Psychiatric patients might be permitted to postpone exams, drop courses, receive special instruction or, if necessary, to take a medical leave of absence or even withdraw from school without academic penalty. For the most part the faculty was very concerned about the students and did not mind a student's return to class at a time when their academic capabilities were significantly impaired. Follow-up psychiatric care was the rule.

It all worked surprisingly well. But how could it work? This was unlike no psychiatric hospital I had ever heard of. I began to ponder on some very unsettling questions.

Where was the psychiatric hospital? What was the psychiatric hospital? What were we really doing?

Inpatient psychiatric treatment at Cowell rested on the assumption that for days to weeks to months before hospitalization the patient had functioned at a level consistent with whatever was required for a person to remain a student at the University. Then something had occurred which had led the patient to decompensate with the appearance of disturbed mood, an impaired grasp of reality, or threatening or self-destructive behavior, along with an inability to function. While the inpatient psychiatric service provided support, comfort and protection, it attempted to help the student patients avoid a persisting regression by pushing them to regain their premorbid level of capability as quickly as possible. The aggressive treatment program began at the time of admission. And the rapid increase in ward privileges and graded passes instituted early in the course of a hospital stay often helped the patients to quickly become their old selves once again.

The University and surrounding community were tolerant of relatively bizarre behavior and dress. No one looked twice at a messy student standing outside a University building shouting at an invisible companion. To some degree this was considered within the realm of normal student behavior. The attitude of the Administration, the faculty, the other students, the police and community as a whole led me to an inescapable conclusion. The psychiatric hospital was potentially the whole campus, with a fluid use of parts of it depending on a patient's condition. The hospital was not a room or a floor of a building. The psychiatric hospital was the area in which the patient's treatment took place with the assistance of as many helpers as possible. The helpers might be health care personnel or friends or faculty or family. At times the hospital was the seclusion room. Other times it was the hospital corridor including the patient's room, the nursing station, and the TV lounge. The psychiatric hospital really could be the entire campus. It could all be configured by the attending psychiatrist to provide an atmosphere for healing psychiatric patients. And the extent to which the hospital resources could be mobilized to conduct the patient's treatment meant doing whatever it took to meet the needs of every patient's condition at any given time.

Six months after I began work on the Cowell inpatient service, Burleigh Kammerer, the chief of the service, resigned. He had decided to devote all of his time to private office practice. On the basis of my level of interest and my performance to date, Saxton Pope asked me to take over as head of the inpatient service. What an opportunity!

This was UC Berkeley with twenty-seven thousand students. Apart from the free speech movement, the sexual revolution, and Vietnam war protest and resistance, this was also the era of the rapid proliferation of drug experimentation. Psychologist Tim Leary was calling for LSD to be put in the drinking water. Some Berkeley therapists were using LSD in misguided attempts at treating patients—even to the point of using it themselves along with their patients. Other hallucinogen use, especially DMT and PCP, became commonplace. We became so busy with treating hallucinogen-related problems that alcohol fell into the background as a treatment issue. We knew that marijuana impaired clear thinking, but it seemed like a minor problem in the face of what became the LSD epidemic.

Of course the problems involving drugs also posed a disruption on campus. One of many students who entered the drug scene, Jay, was a clean cut but totally distraught looking 20-year-old sophomore. He was brought to the emergency room by the police about 1 a.m. because he had caused a loud disturbance in his dormitory.

Jay: "Wow! Wow! Wow!" (shouting, then a pause). "It's coming. I can see it. Beautiful!"

Dr. W: "What are you seeing, Jay?"

Jay: "You know. I've got it! It! It!" (pause) I'm it! I'm part of it. I'm scared! (pause) It's OK. I love it. I'm love!"

Dr. W: "How many dots of acid did you suck?"

Jay: " Four dots! Four dots! Four dots!

Dr. W: "We will help you come out of this, Jay. This is all from the acid. We will help you, and you will be all right."

Jay was given an injection of a mild tranquilizing anti-psychotic drug, Compazine. Within thirty minutes, his level of agitation diminished. After he had calmed to some degree, he was admitted to the hospital. That night he slept about four hours. By the next afternoon he was tired and shaky, but he had no more symptoms of psychosis. His grasp of reality was now intact, and he made sense when he talked. He was discharged back to his dormitory with a supply of Compazine tablets, which he was to take regularly for the next week. Unlike many who have experienced a brief psychotic episode, he did keep his follow-up appointment. At the time he was seen, he showed no signs of serious mental disturbance. But despite what had happened to him, he seemed fascinated with the psychotic experience and flirted with the idea of trying LSD again "perhaps from a better batch."

That was the way it was with LSD. As strange as it seemed, LSD often left the user with the wish to become psychotic again, to have another trip, no matter what the consequences might be.

The campus police and the Berkeley police brought a never-ending stream of drug-impaired, highly disturbed patients to the hospital emergency room. LSD and other hallucinogens drove up the hospital inpatient psychiatric census to a maximum of eighteen patients at a time. The bad trip LSD psychotic patients were typically loud, excited, grandiose, disturbed, scared, and scattered. At times, they were violent. They had elaborate and vivid visual hallucinations and illusions. In addition to the visual distortions, many had auditory hallucinations as well. The voices frequently commanded them to do things.

Because of intense grandiose feelings, many LSD patients believed they were God or had become one with God.

Needless to say, their judgment was profoundly impaired. LSD-inspired delusions that they could fly led students to leap from the roofs of apartment buildings, often with a tragic outcome. If they lived, a number of these students would be left as quadriplegic. Even though paralyzed from the head down, once their medical conditions had stabilized, some of these quadriplegics miraculously were able to return to school. They actually lived at the hospital while they attended classes in their electric wheelchairs.

Fortunately the majority of students with LSD-induced psychosis or anxiety states improved over four to twenty-four hours. They were usually able to return to school within a few days. Most who had had a bad trip did not want to risk recurrence and vowed never to use LSD again despite urges to do so. But some got hooked. The euphoria they had experienced during the LSD trip was a powerful motivator to use LSD again and again.

For a smaller number, the LSD precipitated a schizophrenia-like psychotic illness which was much more resistant to treatment than non-LSD induced schizophrenic illness. Some of this group never got better, their once promising lives now sadly impaired by incurable schizophrenia.

A third group consisted of patients who had had used LSD at least fifteen times. These were regular euphoria seekers who came to a bad end. They developed a different form of psychopathology. They lost ambition. They became unable to focus or concentrate. They had frequent LSD flashbacks during which—without LSD—they experienced "trips," especially bizarre visual distortions. They became much less sensitive to the needs of others, including their own children and other family members. The content of their words was often grandiose, though their voices seemed flattened in tone. They commonly proclaimed that they had a special mission to give LSD to everyone to help them achieve truth and happiness. All dropped out of school and insisted that school or even reading had become irrelevant. This group did not want treatment. I saw some of them for evaluation only because they had been coerced into seeing me by family, friends, or the law.

At age 23, Jerold was married and had a two-year-old son. He was tall, thin, long- haired and poorly groomed and dressed. His body odor was overpowering.

Irritable and suspicious, he had come to my office to "get my wife and family off my back." One year earlier, during his senior year at the University, he had begun what he estimated to be one hundred to two hundred LSD trips. He had dropped out of school.

Dr. W: "Do you plan to go back to school?"
Jerold: "No, man. It was all a waste."
Dr. W: "What do you plan to do?"

Jerold: "I have plans."

Dr. W: "What are they ?"

Jerold: "I'm planning."

Dr. W: "Planning for what? Will you get a job? How will you support your wife and your baby?"

Jerold: "My plans come when I'm in it on the stuff. I have the best plans."

Dr. W: "Do you plan to keep using acid?"

Jerold: "We all should use."

Dr. W: "Do you read any books?"

Jerold: "They don't matter."

After I had interviewed a number of patients like Jerold, I realized that I was looking at young people with some form of persisting, possibly permanent, organic brain damage. Their flashbacks of visual illusions and hallucinations indicated that their retinal rods and cones now had a lowered threshold to stimulation. Their disinterest in reading and learning really was a mere rationalization for the fact that they had lost the ability to learn. I was convinced that they had sustained diffuse frontal, temporal and occipital lobe brain damage as a result of the LSD usage. I did not know to what degree they would recover, or if they would improve at all. What a human tragedy! Here were many bright young people destroying their access to a complete and meaningful life. Some ultimately did make a partial recovery. Others did not.

PCP was an animal tranquilizer now abused by humans. The PCP impacted patients were somewhat similar to the LSD patients except that they were more violent and seemed to possess superhuman strength. If the police report indicated that it had taken four or five officers to subdue the patient, we assumed the culprit drug to have been PCP until proven otherwise.

Over time, my private practice was developing nicely. The inpatient service at Cowell was also operating well. Besides me, three other part-time psychiatrists, two of whom I had recruited and trained, treated patients on the unit. After four years of preparation my Ego Psychology textbook had been accepted for publication. I was happy with the professional part of my life.

During all of this time Berkeley itself had changed, and I did not like it nearly as much. By 1968 the political elements took every excuse to march in the streets, and violent riots ensued—often day after day. For me the crowning blow occurred one day while I was driving my young son home from grade school. "Daddy, look at the monsters!" he exclaimed. He was looking out the window at uniformed members of the National Guard, who at last had arrived to rescue us from violence, anarchy, and the ineptitude of our befuddled city council. The Guard members were wearing gas masks. My son seemed more curious and excited than frightened. But I was the one who was more worried. We were slowly moving through barricades intended to divert traffic from the riot areas. A public address system urged us not to open our car windows lest we be exposed to the effects of tear gas. I wasn't exactly frightened, either; but my heart sank heavily in my chest. I felt very guilty and regretful. This was no way to bring up children. What kind of a father was I? I had to get my family out of Berkeley as soon as I could.

My family's escape from Berkeley took longer than I had hoped. In the fall of 1968 I got a big surprise!

XIII. THE DOCTOR'S SURPRISE

Good surprises are usually small—such as getting a raise or bonus when none had been anticipated, or a gift you had hoped for but didn't really expect. Big surprises are very different. They tend to fall into the category of bad news. One day a surprise of the big bad news variety appeared in my mail. It was a notice from my draft board. I hadn't heard from them in years, and I knew any word from them wasn't going to be good. The unexpected letter I held in my hand loudly announced that I had been drafted! At age thirty-four and one half, I had been conscripted into the military.

My draft board and I had had a long standing, very distant relationship. I never saw any members of the draft board. But whoever and whereever they were, they seemed to have been stalking me for many years. As the law had then required, I initially registered for the draft at age eighteen. Over time I received a number of deferments from being drafted—first for being a college student, then for being a medical student, and later for being married with children. This time my argument that I had three small children and a large private practice in psychiatry did not seem to matter at all. The University of California administration protested to my draft board something to the effect that I alone protected the whole population at UC Berkeley from becoming floridly psychotic.

Surprisingly nothing could be done. My appeals were like throwing messages in corked bottles into a stormy sea. No last minute reprieve reversed my having been drafted. The country was at war in Vietnam, and doctors were needed. A special draft for doctors up to age thirty-five had recently been enacted, and at thirty-four and a half, I was a prime candidate. I passed a perfunctory physical exam (which no conscripted physician ever had failed). Chronic bronchial asthma and flat feet did not matter. An FBI background check and a personal interview gave me a security clearance. Having attended Young Socialist League beer parties in college or having an old membership in Fair Play for Cuba had no impact. Undoubtedly I was wanted, and nothing whatever was going to prevent my being in the military.

All conscripted doctors automatically were destined for the Army. That meant boot camp was only weeks away from the time I opened my "greetings" from the draft board letter. But I had been drafted because I was a doctor. What good was to come of my going to boot camp? Avoiding boot camp was possible only if I were to enlist in one of the other military services. I began a frantic series of phone calls to Washington to talk to anyone in the Navy or the Air Force bureaucracy who might have any interest in me. The Navy liked what I had to offer. I seemed to fit into their needs. And the Navy miraculously fit into mine! They made a wonderful proposal. My new job as a US Navy officer was to direct the psychiatric residency training program at the Oakland Naval Hospital, a twenty minute drive from my home in Berkeley. The Navy also planned that I run a psychiatric inpatient unit for the treatment of officers and military dependents. I would not have to sell my home or leave my family. Incredibly I would not even have to give up my private practice. After 4:30 p.m. and on weekends they told me I was free to see my private practice patients.

That early morning when I arrived at the Oakland Naval Hospital, Oak Knoll, I was informed that the following day I would begin a two week training course to teach me basic military fundamentals. I was supposed to learn how to dress properly in a military uniform, how to salute, how to march, and even how to address others in the military. Ed Morhauser, the psychiatric resident who had been in charge of the unit I was to direct, was both happy and relieved to see me. He announced that he was scheduled to leave for vacation that afternoon and wanted no delay in his departure. Within hours of my arrival, the unit was to be left to me. Because of the urgent need to have me run the unit, the nursing staff received permission from Vic Holm, the head of the Oak Knoll psychiatric service, for my orientation course to be postponed. Yet the staff made it clear that they did not want to be embarrassed or disgraced by some hick who knew nothing about military protocol. Within fifteen minutes after I had arrived on the unit, they had appropriately rearranged my newly purchased uniform and taught me how to salute passably if not properly. Their nonstop laughter confirmed my suspicion that I looked silly. I felt like a not yet housebroken puppy. Reinforced by the dictate of the head of the department, the staff insisted that I learn very quickly how to at least pretend to look and act like an officer. And by the end of the first day I had a superficial and uncomfortable familiarity with my new role. Over the next two years, because the demands of the unit took all of my time, I never did get to take the basic military orientation course.

I was not the only newly arrived conscripted psychiatrist. A half-dozen others were there, all age thirty-four and all somewhat stunned at having been plucked out of junior faculty positions at different medical schools. While some were angry at the disruption of their lives, all were relieved to have awakened in California. Other drafted psychiatrists were being sent to Vietnam or to hospital ships off the coast of Vietnam. We got to meet some of them while they were home on leave from their duty stations. While we felt sorry for them, we were quietly grateful that we were not the ones to be going out there.

The Oak Knoll group of psychiatrists was very talented, and the combination proved electric. While they had all been faculty members at different medical schools, they represented many schools of thought in psychiatry. And the next two years were filled with spirited discussion and often heated argument as we attempted to convince one another of what we each knew to be truth in psychiatry. All of us came away wiser for the effort. It seemed amazing how many changes were taking place in our field. And Oak Knoll had become the unique place where all of these changes could be discussed and tested. This was by far the most talented hospital medical staff that I could recall. The psychiatric residents training there at Oak Knoll were keenly aware that something unique was happening right around them, and that they stood to gain tremendously from studying with a star studded faculty.

The department head, Vic Holm, was a career navy psychiatrist. He was solid; he radiated integrity. An excellent administrator, he wisely recognized that he had been endowed with a dream team of gifted players. He coached lightly from the side-lines—always permitting his superstars to display their clinical and teaching talents.

At the time I arrived at Oak Knoll, all of the psychiatric hospital units were housed in run down World War II Quonset huts. One month later a brand new high-rise hospital tower opened fifty yards away. It was a lovely state of the art hospital, and we moved into modern well-designed quarters. While the setting had changed overnight from Quonset huts to a brand new facility, my previous experience at San Francisco General and at Cowell Hospital at UC Berkeley had taught me that the physical plant of the hospital itself did not really matter in our quest to provide better and better treatment. It was clearer than ever that a psychiatric hospital was less of a defined place and more of a concept. At Berkeley the 'hospital' was flexible and had ranged from a patient's room to the whole University campus.

I realized that a psychiatric hospital was like a machine for fixing people. It was up to us, the medical staff, to design that machine to recognize and fix each patient's broken parts. I could now put it all together and make it work without interference. My rank in the military structure as Lieutenant Commander and later as full Commander guaranteed me the authority that I needed. This was no University of Chicago Psychiatric service where my presence as a medical school student was part of a teaching game. This was no Manteno State Hospital where few staff or patients had any hope for change. This was no San Francisco General Hospital where I had to struggle with a narrow minded director at a time when I was just beginning to understand what a psychiatric hospital was all about. And this was no UC Berkeley where I had to share the staff and most of the treatment space with internists and surgeons.

Why should anyone be in a psychiatric hospital? Why should anyone be placed involuntarily in a psychiatric unit? Just what was a psychiatric hospital supposed to do for a troubled person? The essence of the psychiatric hospital, as I had now come to see it, was a series of functions. The psychiatric hospital was a shelter, a place to be safe from the world, safe from one's own self destructive behavior, safe from one's own aggressive or violent behavior, and safe from being driven by one's own intense cravings for drugs or alcohol. It was also a place to feel secure, accepted and understood; a place to resurrect hope and to eliminate despair; a place that offered intensive treatment to help heal as quickly as possible. It was a place to pause, a respite to recover from intense painful feelings elicited at work or at home. It was a place to come back to reality; a place that provided the reassurance of order and structure. It was a place that evaluated and treated medical problems that might be determining or complicating behavior or intense feelings. It was a place for a patient to take a crash course in developing skills for dealing with family, peers, work, oneself and the world in general.

If this was what a psychiatric hospital was supposed to do, some types of psychiatric hospital were far less effective than others in achieving these goals. It now seemed clear that not all types of psychiatric hospitals were up to the job.

Manteno State Hospital had been a warehouse. Most state hospitals I had read about or subsequently visited were little better. The function of the warehouse was less to provide treatment than to keep the seriously ill patients in the closet and away from the rest of the community. The closure of most of the state hospitals beginning in the 1960s resulted in hordes of homeless mentally ill patients wandering around the urban centers of many American cities. The majority of these street people are treatable but actively refuse or resist treatment. Efforts to provide involuntary treatment are Herculean and expensive, and the majority of community programs seriously aimed at helping those patients become exhausted and give up.

On the other hand, many patients do get by in the community. They have improved to the point where they can live in board and care homes and participate in some outpatient community programs. The advent and widespread use of psychiatric medication has made this transformation possible.

Other models of psychiatric hospitals all had serious drawbacks. In the University model too much time was spent evaluating patients, and the delay in initiating aggressive treatment had led to regression and the road to chronic mental illness.

The "Doctor Does It" model of treatment pretended that the patient never talked meaningfully to anyone else except to the doctor. In this model the doctors were supposed to provide all of the treatment—whether it be the patient's psychotherapy or the initiation of different organic approaches. The only function of the hospital staff was to provide three decent meals, clean linen and reasonable amusement between doctor visits. Hospital staff members were often forbidden to take part in the treatment provided by the doctor, and at times doctors did not even tell the staff what was going on with the patient. It was left to the staff to puzzle it out, if they even cared to try.

But in reality the doctor was not always pivotal in a patient's hospital treatment. Patients spent most of their time with the staff and in most instances very much wanted to talk with them. For example, one patient told me that what helped her the most was having coffee each afternoon with a dietary worker who reminded her of her warm and loving grandmother. The "doctor does it" model made the staff want to give up. It wasted their potential for implementing detailed individualized treatment plans.

By contrast, even the county hospital "Revolving Door" model looked pretty good. This model relied heavily on staff involvement. A team approach was critical. Rapidly formulated treatment plans were the rule. The problem with the county hospital model was the economically-driven pressure to turn patients out of the hospital prematurely to make room for others. Even seriously ill patients had to be discharged before they had improved enough to be able to benefit from treatment at a less intensive level of care. Premature discharge all too often led to suicide, violence or repeated flare-ups of psychosis.The revolving door model fostered the development of chronic long term mental illness.

The serious defects of all of these models provided lessons about what should be included in an optimally effective psychiatric hospital. Now was the time to make good on a pledge I had made while still a medical student after I had left Manteno State Hospital. At the time I had pledged to myself and to anyone who was willing to listen that a better psychiatric hospital could be developed. Oak Knoll was going to be that opportunity.

The principles now seemed fairly simple and clear.

An effective psychiatric hospital should institute treatment as soon as a patient is admitted. Even if the treatment plan were wrong (and it usually was not wrong), it could always be changed as long as there was a mechanism for frequent review of each patient's progress. The treatment plan would be undertaken by all of the treatment staff who regularly talked to one another about their ongoing observations and suggestions. Staff members' talking insured they were on the same page regarding each patient's treatment. In this model patients would have to be hospitalized long enough so that progress was sustainable, with a lower probability of regression after discharge.

Each patient's ego function defects were clearly identified at the time of admission to the hospital. For example, one patient might have a defective grasp of reality with delusions and hallucinations. Another might have a problem with self-destructive impulses, possibly intent on suicide. A third might be troubled by confused thinking. Still another might have difficulty controlling waves of intense angry feelings in response to minor stress. If the patient's symptoms and behavior were seen as a series of ego weaknesses, the hospital through its programs now implemented by its staff attempted to strengthen and bolster those specific defects by 'loaning' the patients some of the ego strengths of the staff members. As the treatment progressed, the patient's defective ego functions became stronger.

At Oak Knoll I now had the ultimate authority and responsibility for producing positive results. And I was determined that all patients on my unit were going to get well.

After my first day on the unit, the shock of being transformed from a civilian doctor into a Navy officer had passed. The next morning I met with the charge nurse, Beverly Collins, and the rest of my unit staff to begin teaching them about the treatment program I planned to install. I explained what we were going to do, and why we were going to do it. We would meet as a treatment team five mornings per week to review the state of the unit. We would examine each patient's medical record to share information about patient progress or lack thereof and explain and upgrade the treatment plan. I would elaborate each staff member's role in implementing treatment plans. Afterward, on three days each week we as a team would proceed to bedside doctors rounds. I briefly interviewed every patient and demonstrated to the staff the kind of psychotherapeutic interaction that might be most helpful. Some of the staff learned how to effectively conduct bedside interviews.

A community meeting for all patients and staff took place daily after doctor's rounds and at the same time on other days when there were no doctor's rounds. The community meetings were chaired by a psychiatric resident or a nurse. These meetings were a form of group therapy. Each patient was addressed within the framework of his individual treatment plan. The staff also attempted to teach patients how to interact with one another. The intent was that patients, too, should take part in one another's treatment plans. After the community meetings the staff and resident had 'feedback' sessions to review what had transpired. Unless restricted to the unit for specific therapeutic reasons, patients then went off to the occupational therapy area. As much as possible the occupational therapist translated each patient's treatment plan into occupational therapy activities. These occupational therapy activities ranged from group projects to conventional arts and crafts to weight lifting to games to cooking and baking. After lunch, patients had some free time. In the afternoons the staff led talks and discussions often featuring current events or cognitive therapy or information about psychiatric drugs. In the evening, patients and staff had a 'wrap up' group session to talk about what had happened during the day, including whether there were any issues of concern to the ward. Some patients used these meetings to discuss problems bound to arise when very different types of people live together in a relatively small space. Other patients talked about their progress or their problems. Sometime during the course of each day, all patients met with their doctors for individual therapy sessions.

The intent of all this structured activity was to shape the patient's environment up to twenty-four hours per day. Each patient could have a number of therapeutically tailored experiences that would enable him to benefit from his individualized treatment plan.

The staff liked being let in on the action of treating patients. They appreciated learning what to do, and understanding why they were doing it. They shared in the satisfaction that comes from watching patients improve day by day, and knowing that they were an important part of the treatment.

Here is an example of how it worked:

Some voices were obviously more real to patients than other voices, and it was our task to help them grasp which was which. "Of course I hear voices," Lyle assured us. "I've heard them for years. Doesn't everyone? It is God's voice telling me what to do. God told me to punch out the windows. And I did it."

In our new approach to treatment our job was not to try to find out if God's voice resembled the voice of Lyle's autocratic one time naval officer father. Our task was for us to stand for reality so as to help Lyle improve his own grasp of reality.

When we talked to Lyle, the staff and I all said essentially the same thing. "You don't really hear God's voice. You do hear voices, but they are not real. They seem very real to you right now, but the voices are symptoms of your illness. You have a type of schizophrenia, and hearing voices is a common symptom of that illness. We are going to help you to get rid of the voices."

All of the staff would repeat this message in many daily encounters with the patient. In the group therapy community meetings, we would suggest to other patients that they join us in similar interactions with Lyle. We commonly gave families the same type of instruction in helping them to deal with a psychotic family member.

During the two years that I worked at Oak Knoll, the hospital 'fixed' people almost all of the time. Patients received excellent care and improved significantly. Many even got well. The psychiatric residents and the nursing staff learned more than they ever expected. A number were inspired to go on to have distinguished careers in psychiatry. The Navy administration was immensely pleased with the high quality of psychiatric service we provided.

Toward the end of my tenure in the Navy I was asked to present a talk on how everything worked and why it all worked so well. At the end of the talk one of the residents, Gene Voltolina, said, "Wow! Is that what we were doing all of this time?" Vic Holm became tearful when I was discharged. The charge nurse, Beverly Collins, a therapeutic zealot in her own right, left the military service at the same time that I did and later became head nurse at several facilities where I had clinical administrative positions. One of my most talented residents, Steve Heisler, later became my trusted partner in practice and in operating psychiatric hospitals.

Whatever diverse personal opinions the psychiatric faculty might have had about the Vietnam War were largely kept private when we were at work at the hospital. When away from the hospital, we were more outspoken. I could always count on being denounced as a fascist if I went to a Berkeley cocktail party wearing my officer's uniform. Then, as now, the same university community that was eager to endorse the Free Speech Movement was intolerant of any dissent from its politically correct views.

But in my work I knew that I was helping military officers, many of whom were deeply affected by what they had experienced in combat. And I felt good knowing that, along with the rest of the conscripted faculty, I was helping train another generation of psychiatrists for their careers as clinicians. I hoped that the quality of their education would enable them to emerge at the cutting edge of the field.

XIV. LOBOTOMY IN THE BASEMENT

She had always seemed emotional and a trifle prone to exaggeration. Yet I knew Dr Graham was a good psychiatrist. Today at a department of psychiatry meeting she was her usual volatile self, except even a bit more so. "Lobotomies are being performed in the basement of this hospital!" she shouted. She said she had been tipped off by a late night phone call from a frightened and distraught nursing staff member whose name she had sworn not to divulge. The poor nurse had been commanded to assist in the procedure and feared loss of her job for whistle-blowing.

The psychiatric staff at Herrick Memorial Hospital, Berkeley, California, met monthly. It was commonplace for people to say off the wall and seemingly stupid things at these meetings. All in all the meetings were boring and inconsequential. I often wondered if I should continue to attend.

At the time of her outburst, all I could think of was how absurd Graham's charges sounded. She had often made loud and totally groundless accusations aimed at the hospital administrator or other members of the medical staff. Surely this must be another of her drama queen fantasies or nightmares.

After all, we were living in 1970, and lobotomy was almost universally considered barbaric and immoral. Wasn't lobotomy a kind of execution of the soul, a process for the permanent destruction of creativity, the capacity for fun and solid intellective thinking— leaving behind a dull robot-like shell of a subhuman? I hadn't even heard about lobotomy for years. Yet here was Dr. Graham proclaiming that lobotomies were being done secretly in our very own hospital, the place where we doctors were treating our patients every day. She insisted that patients were often transferred from the psychiatric service to the surgical service where they were then lobotomized. And none of us at the psychiatric staff meeting knew that this was happening!

But if it were true, someone on the psychiatric staff had to know about it. Some one or possibly more than one of us psychiatrists, possibly someone or more of us at the meeting, must actually be referring patients for lobotomy. "Who on this staff is referring patients for lobotomy? And who is the lobotomist?" I asked. Graham said that she didn't know. No one in the room confessed or dared to volunteer a guess.

And if lobotomies were being done, certainly the hospital administrator must know.

Furthermore, if in fact there were a lobotomist, who was he? Was he one of the handful of neurosurgeons on the hospital staff whom we saw daily in the doctor's lounge or at medical staff meetings? Was it someone else?

That it could be someone else was unlikely but vaguely possible. The hospital medical staff bylaws had a provision which said that under certain special circumstances the hospital administrator was able to grant temporary privileges to doctors not on the medical staff. But for lobotomy? It all seemed beyond belief.

Herrick Memorial Hospital was an acute care general hospital located less than a mile from the University of California Berkeley campus. The hospital had a large inpatient psychiatric service. My private practice office was located directly across the street from the hospital. After I had been discharged from the Navy, I devoted most of my time to building my practice. I really enjoyed helping very sick patients whose severity of illness often mandated intensive psychiatric hospital care. It was convenient for me to take care of my hospitalized patients at Herrick.

The majority of the patients admitted to the hospital psychiatric service were treated by one particular group of four psychiatrists who were well known in the community. The members of this group considered the psychiatric units to be their personal fiefdom. They regarded the rest of us psychiatrists who tried to treat patients at the hospital as intruders into their royal preserve. Because they admitted so many patients, the favored group had a special relationship with the hospital administrator. They dictated policy, and the administrator listened. There was no doubt that the regal group had special privilege. And the rest of us justifiably felt downtrodden. If the psychiatric units were crowded, patients of the favored group on the waiting list for admission routinely bypassed the names of patients of the other psychiatrists.

Doctors outside of the royal group had little say about what went on regarding the treatment programs or the operation of the psychiatric units. The monthly psychiatric staff meetings gave the non-royal doctors a platform to talk about what we thought should be done to improve the service. Most of the time we were venting to one another, and our suggestions rarely left the room. Members of the royal group opted not to attend the monthly staff meetings. A junior administration member took notes but said almost nothing. We thought of her as an administration spy.

When Graham made the charge of lobotomy in our hospital, there was a general sense of outrage. Those of us present at the meeting quietly suspected that, if there were any truth to the charge, it must be the royal group of psychiatrists whose patients were being referred for lobotomy. But no one at the meeting had the courage to say anything outright. A public accusation might result in the accuser having a hard time getting his patients

admitted into the hospital for treatment. Since everyone present knew that the royal group and, to a lesser
degree, the administration didn't like me anyway, I was
volunteered to be part of a three-person committee
appointed to investigate the lobotomy issue. We were to
report back in a month. After the staff meeting the other
two designated committee members became very nervous about their charge and backed off, using a variety
of nonsensical excuses. One remembered he was going
on a vacation. The other felt his practice was already
overloaded, and that he couldn't give the project the
time it deserved. They were happy to name me as the
sole investigator.

The royal group had reason to dislike me. It was clear
to them that amongst the junior psychiatric staff at the
hospital there was movement for change in the ways
patients were being treated. And all too often I was the
spokesman for proposed change.

Regardless of their dislike, I contacted a senior member of the dominant psychiatric group and asked him
point blank if there were any truth to the rumors about
lobotomy being performed at our hospital. He didn't
sound the least bit surprised. I guessed that he knew I was
coming. He must have had advance warning through
the administration spy who had sat in on the psychiatric staff meeting. He readily acknowledged that he
and other members of his group often referred patients
for lobotomy. These were usually patients who had not
responded to electric shock treatment. He believed that

some patients who were tortured by obsessive depressive thoughts were made much more comfortable by lobotomy. His tone was arrogant. Clearly he felt comfortable in the fact that his group had full control over the administrator of the hospital.

He even gave me the name of the lobotomist, Dr Charles Freeman. I was puzzled. Freeman was not a member of the regular Herrick Hospital medical staff. How could he in essence 'sneak' into the hospital and lobotomize patients? I was told that Freeman had been granted "temporary privileges" by the administration. Most hospitals had medical staff bylaws which contained a provision that a physician, not a member of the regular medical staff, could under certain unusual conditions and in the judgment of the chief of staff or the administrator of the hospital be granted temporary privileges to help in the treatment of some single patient. But to have this provision used in such a loose way was far from what most of us envisioned as its real intent. Freeman was being given total license to operate at Herrick Hospital on as many patients as were referred his way.

I phoned Freeman the following day. Was this the same Charles Freeman who had written articles about the thousands of lobotomies he had performed in state hospitals in New York or Pennsylvania or Ohio? Freeman was not the least bit surprised at my call. Clearly he had been briefed about my checking out what was going on. I was the surprised one when Freeman invited me to watch him perform a lobotomy. Of course I agreed, although I had to suppress feelings of revulsion at the same time. My charge as an investigator mandated that I get at the truth, even if it meant attending a lobotomy. I felt like an undercover agent being invited to watch a gang member murder.

Charles Freeman was famous—or more appropriately, he was infamous. He had performed nearly 3500 loboto-mies in 23 states. He was a neurologist with some surgical training. As an assistant to a famous neurosurgeon in 1936, he had begun lobotomizing patients. At the time the procedure was laborious and lengthy, involving the standard many hour craniotomy procedure of sawing a bone flap in a patient's skull to gain access to his brain. At most one or two procedures could be performed on any given day.

But it was Freeman alone who invented a much faster and more effective way of performing lobotomies. Originally he used an ordinary ice pick. Later he modified the ice pick into a an instrument called a leucotome, designed specifically for the lobotomy procedure.

Freeman became an evangelist for lobotomy, envisioning that large populations could be treated quickly and simply. He embarked on a national campaign in his van, which he called the "lobotomobile," to demonstrate his technique to other doctors, especially those working in large state mental hospitals. Freeman would show off his procedure by ice picking both of a patient's eye sockets at one time—one ice pick in each hand.

The operating room seemed dark except for the brilliant lights that beamed down upon a sad looking dazed middle-aged woman who was restrained to a large leather chair. The chair itself looked like it had been borrowed from a dentist's office. Even had she been motivated, there was no possibility for escape.

According to Freeman she had a history of multiple episodes of severe depression which in the past had responded to a course of electric shock treatments. But each new episode of depression had responded more poorly to a new course of electric shock.

Freeman explained that the current procedure for lobotomy was really quite easy. The old procedure had involved lifting up a triangle of bone in the skull. Then under full direct vision of the brain, the neurosurgeon had severed some of the tracts that connected the frontal lobes with the brain's emotion centers. It had all been elaborate and time consuming. The new procedure, he explained, was really wonderful and very fast. The whole operation took about ten minutes. If there were enough patients who "required" the procedure, he was able to perform twenty to forty lobotomies per day. Patients recovered quickly and could be discharged home within forty-eight hours after surgery.

The operating room seemed very dark with only a few brilliant lights illuminating center stage. The patient sat motionless, attended by Freeman and a silent operating room nurse, whom I suspected was the agonized whistle-blower who had tipped off Dr Graham. The

lobotomy candidate was given an intravenous anesthetic followed by succinyl choline, a powerful muscle
relaxant related to curare. She was then given an electric shock treatment, the effect of which was scarcely
noticeable because of the anesthetic and muscle relaxant. Freeman explained that this was all the anesthesia
that was required. He then inserted a curved retractor
around the top of the patient's right eyeball and moved
the whole eye slightly downward. Over the top of the
eye he inserted the ice pick-like leucotome. When he
felt the instrument was properly positioned with its point
against the thin bone at the back of the orbit just behind
the eyeball, he took a small mallet and gently tapped
on the bottom of the leucotome. After a few taps, the
stiletto-like instrument popped through the back of the
orbit and into the right frontal lobe of the brain. Freeman
inserted the leucotome to a set depth. He then used the
entry point through the back of the orbit as a fulcrum,
and he moved the dermatome up and down, creating a fan shaped cut in the brain tissue. After giving the
patient a second electric shock, he repeated the procedure on the other side. As promised, the whole operation
took less than ten minutes. "All she will have tomorrow will
be black eyes and a headache. She won't remember a
thing," said Freeman. The only complication of doing the
procedure this way was the rare possibility of cutting a
major cerebral artery. If that happened, then the patient
would have to undergo an emergency life saving craniotomy. Freeman boasted that this happened very rarely.

I could scarcely believe how quickly the whole pro-cedure had taken place. Up to now I had wondered at the psychiatric literature describing the results of thou-sands of lobotomies performed at several East Coast state hospitals. It finally all made sickening sense. Using the leucotome procedure, an energetic surgeon could lobotomize large numbers of patients in almost no time at all.

I envisioned corridors lined with benches occupied by heavily sedated men and women clad in gray hospital gowns. As each person's name or number was called, two attendants provided escort through swinging doors into the surgery. The solid wood doors with clouded glass windows obscured the chamber where, with a few quick taps and fan shaped swings of the leucotome, the patient's soul disappeared. The leucotome was the tool of the executioner masquerading in the gown of a surgeon.

I politely thanked Freeman for permitting me to be an observer. Inside I wanted to wretch. But it had all been like a surreal dream. Watching the lobotomy reminded me of my first unbelievable days at Manteno State Hospital back in 1956. Yet here we were in 1970! Just before I left the operating room, Freeman said, "Just don't put me out of business." I did not answer. I knew my charge.

My charge was to study lobotomy at our hospi-tal, to do an in-depth review of the scientific literature about lobotomy, and to report back to my committee. Of course my real goal was to put a stop to lobotomy.

I vary much wanted to put Freeman out of business. The committee had asked me to write a report of my findings, which would be presented at the next department of psychiatry meeting.

To complete my report, I did an elaborate literature review. I even read a Jesuit volume, "Ethics of Psychosurgery." I confess that I had started my investigation with the determination that I would prevent more lobotomies from being performed at Herrick Hospital. But after my literature review, I came to the surprising conclusion that lobotomy, as horrible as it was, theoretically could be valuable on very rare occasions—when no other method provided relief. But since the many new psychiatric drugs given alone or in combination made the prospect for improvement or cure ever so much better, the likelihood of having to resort to lobotomy had become almost infinitesimal.

The department of psychiatry adopted my report. They recommended that while lobotomy was an extreme procedure, it might be indicated in some cases. But there would have to be a procedure for control of its use. Approval for lobotomy would require the unanimous vote of a panel of three psychiatrists, none of whom was the patient's treating doctor. I felt that a reasoned and objective approach had prevailed.

What subsequently happened was that no patient was ever referred to the panel. The regal group knew that approval for lobotomy by a panel of three independent psychiatrists on the staff would never be forthcoming.

And as a result no other lobotomies were performed at Herrick Hospital. The need to comply with the approval procedure was one of the limiting factors.

The other factor that put a stop to lobotomy was Herrick Hospital's location in Berkeley and the threat of exposure. I had casually talked to one of the charge nurses about my vision of the hospital and some of its clinicians appearing in investigatory newspaper articles describing patient care atrocities. All it would take would be one or two phone calls. It took little imagination to foresee TV cameras in front of the hospital along with hundreds of student marchers bearing placards and chanting, "Killers! Killers!" I knew my musings would be relayed to the administrator. The prospect of exposure in the papers and on TV was so frightening to the administration that despite the clout of the dominant psychiatric group, lobotomy at Herrick Hospital was stopped forever.

XV. NEW HOPE
IN THE BURBS

By 1972 the proliferation of psychiatric inpatient benefits as part of health insurance made it much more possible to treat large numbers of the mentally ill who previously could not have afforded private mental health care. The use of psychiatric drugs had became so effective that patients' lengths of stay in psychiatric hospitals were dramatically shorter than the interminable state hospital incarcerations of the past. Many patients who once would have been hospitalized could by this time avoid hospitalization altogether and were treatable on an outpatient basis. Once hospital lengths of stay became relatively brief, insurance companies could afford to bet that any given person would never require psychiatric hospitalization, or that psychiatric hospital care, if needed, would be finite in time and in cost.

Now that insurance payment for psychiatric hospital treatment was available, the prospect of profit led to the massive growth of the psychiatric hospital indus-try. The decision to build a new psychiatric hospital in the suburb of Walnut Creek was made by Community Psychiatric Centers, a publicly owned psychiatric hos-pital company, as part of its overall development. The company's aggressive expansion plan was to build five new psychiatric hospitals per year strategically placed to maximize utilization by patients whose health insur-ance plans would include inpatient psychiatric cover-age. Walnut Creek was one of the suburbs that fit into the company's master plan for growth.

Located only ten miles east of Berkeley, Walnut Creek seemed to be on a different planet. Almost every house and every building was new and sparkling. Cornfields and orchards of walnut trees were being swept away by massive tract home development and a greatly expanded, mostly brand-new downtown.

In 1972 one of those cornfields was to become a sixty-six bed psychiatric hospital, Walnut Creek Hospital. At first it was only a rumor. To me even the rumor of a psy-chiatric hospital to be built in Walnut Creek seemed like the escape from Berkeley I had often dreamed about. At Herrick Hospital, the fiefdom of the royal group of psy-chiatrists, there was no chance of developing a hospital treatment system that could provide the optimal patient care that I knew to be possible. The existing system, developed to please the royal group, was cast in con-crete. And in my efforts to bring about positive change

I always felt like I was smashing my head against that concrete set of walls.

Walnut Creek Hospital might provide an opportunity for creating a first rate psychiatric hospital. When I first phoned Community Psychiatric Centers' home office in Southern California to inquire about the planned hospital, I was surprised that Jim Conte, the president of the company, wanted to talk to me. He had already heard of me. But what he had heard was a negative report provided by the royal group at Herrick. It was the royal group that had invited CPC to look into the feasibility of a psychiatric hospital in Walnut Creek. CPC had already committed to provide free office space for the royal group if they would shift a large portion of their practice to the new hospital.

Despite the negative report from the royal group, Conte wanted to meet me. I was flattered that he wanted to meet at my office. He instantly struck me as polished, brilliant and hard. I was certain that his business suit cost more than a thousand dollars. He also wore a thin layer of charm like the painted veneer of a piece of cheap furniture. His words were clipped and his tone studied. They carried the aura of insincerity that we most commonly endure in politicians repeating their canned campaign speeches. While I felt he was not a man anyone could trust, he held what might be the key to my future. I knew I would have to deal with him despite any of my reservations about his character.

He seemed impressed with my track record and with my ideas for developing and operating a state of the art psychiatric hospital. After we had talked for awhile, he said that I seemed like I would be a good medical director for the new hospital. I felt a burst of euphoria. But my excitement was suddenly deflated when he added that my becoming the medical director at Walnut Creek Hospital was to be contingent on my receiving the blessing of the royal group. If I were going to become the medical director, this was a chance to show my skills. He explained that I would have to work with the royal group at the new hospital. They had promised Conte that they were going to admit a large number of patients to the new hospital, and I needed at least their pledge that we were going to get along. It seemed like an impossible prerequisite. The royal group hated me. At Herrick Hospital I had been the champion of the faction of young psychiatrists who were challenging their control of the psychiatric service. They would never agree to my being in a position at any hospital which gave me authority to monitor or influence the care they provided patients.

I had little hope. Nonetheless I met with the head of the royal group. His sharp rodent-like stare always made me nervous. I expected to be bitten at any moment. Doing my best to conceal my almost paranoid suspicions, I tried to look friendly and sincere. Before he said much of anything, I told him frankly that I wanted the medical directorship of the new hospital. I promised that if we worked under the same roof at what was to be called Walnut Creek Hospital, I would respect his group's style of treatment.

His response surprised me. He said he was uncertain as to whether Walnut Creek Hospital, a gamble off in the undeveloped suburbs, would be successful at all. His group was well established and relatively happy at Herrick. He confessed that he and other members of his group had no immediate plans to move their practices to what they saw as a risky effort. They might hospitalize a few patients at the new hospital if it seemed convenient for them, but that was all. He added that he and his group would be happier still if I were out of Herrick Hospital and banished to the suburbs. I happily agreed to stay away from Herrick once the new hospital opened if he gave me his group's endorsement.

Even his lukewarm endorsement was good enough for Conte, and I became the medical director for a psychiatric hospital barely under construction. I had asked Conte for very little except the authority to make the hospital the best that it could possibly be, a modest salary and an incentive contract. The contract to which we agreed looked good from both sides. A small salary plus ten per cent of no or little profit looked like a great deal for Conte. For me a small salary plus ten per cent of some profit with no upside cap looked exciting. I was especially keen on a proviso that I be given the freedom to run the hospital without canned company programs as long as the hospital made money. I also had insisted that I retain authority to hire all clinical department heads. Recalling her success at Oak Knoll, I hired Beverly Collins as the Director of Nursing, one of the key positions for the success of any hospital.

Once it had been completed, the hospital looked more like a new modern resort motel than it did a hospital. It was an olive colored one-story wood frame building that came close to surrounding a large grass courtyard. Loosely attached were an administration building and a building that housed the cafeteria, the occupational therapy craft shop and several additional offices. The whole property was beautifully landscaped with green lawns, a variety of bushes and trees, and a lovely fountain near the entrance to the grounds. The interior of the building consisted of two functional units, each subdivided into a locked high security austerely furnished section, and an unlocked section whose wood imitation plastic furniture resembled a Ramada Inn. The beauty disguised the effective function of the physical plant. While every room had large picture windows looking out at lawns or farm houses, all of the windows were made of high security Plexiglas. Chairs thrown at the windows by escape minded patients bounced harmlessly back to the would be escapee whose elopement plan had just been foiled. I surmised that it might be easier to escape through a wall than through a window.

On opening day to get things going, I transferred five of my patients from Herrick Hospital. Within a few days other patients were admitted by some of the psychiatrists who already had established practices in the Walnut Creek area. Since there had been no psychiatric hospital in the immediate area before, none of them had treated hospitalized patients for a number of years. Most didn't have a clue as to how to treat a patient in a psychiatric hospital. Each of these charter psychiatrists had at best a few of his own ideas. Almost none of them liked having their work with patients reviewed at multidisciplinary case conferences five days a week. They all tended to operate on the "Doctor Does It" model. They did not want the staff to participate in their patients' treatment. They felt affronted when I or other members of the hospital staff asked them questions or made suggestions regarding the diagnosis, treatment or management of their patients. Many of these charter doctors were not very capable clinicians, and their wishes to avoid review of their work may have had something to do with fear of exposure. One proved himself so inept that within three months after the hospital opened, he was forced to resign by a committee of his peers. He had prescribed a medication at sixteen times its customary dosage. The nursing staff recognized that the patient's life would be in jeopardy, and they refused to give the patient the lethal dose that had been prescribed.

Over a period of a few years I recruited a new young medical staff who quickly replaced most of the charter medical staff. The new medical staff members were mostly fresh out of residency training programs. They were much sharper than the charter doctors. For the most part they were able to work as team players. They needed the hospital as a source of patients for their practices. And the hospital, as a result of its marketing programs, generated large numbers of referrals for them.

One day I received a call from a psychiatrist, Dr. Alonza Johnson, inquiring whether there might be an opportunity for him to work at Walnut Creek Hospital. I told him that there could be such an opportunity, and I invited him to visit the hospital. He then bluntly said, "I'm black. Do you have any prejudice against black doctors? Is Walnut Creek Hospital a white man's club?" I told him we were only prejudiced against bad doctors. If he were a bad doctor, then we did not want him. We met, and he joined the staff. Johnson was an outstanding clinician. He knew how a psychiatric hospital could work, and he had high expectations for clinical outcomes, no matter how sick a patient might be. I was always pleased to hear his ideas during the daily case conferences.

The hospital was a success almost from the beginning. The treatment programs worked well, and patients improved. We determined to let the whole world know that we had the world's best psychiatric treatment program. We wanted everyone to visit Walnut Creek Hospital and to talk with us about how we treated patients. Invitations went to physicians of all disciplines, psychiatrists, psychologists, social workers, therapists, clergy, hospital administrators, county health professionals, politicians, board and care operators, law enforcement personnel, and the public at large. We invited anyone who might come. And they did come—in numbers far greater than I had ever expected.Visitors came for breakfasts, lunches, or dinners—all with tours and talks. I told my staff, "We want a greater number of visitors to Walnut Creek Hospital than the number of people who visit Disneyland." Of course we did not reach those grandiose numbers, but we did get plenty of visitors. More important, the visitors ended up referring us droves of patients

I hired young, energetic, therapeutic zealots as clinical department heads and staff. We taught them a good deal about flexible, highly individualized treatment planning. They saw amazing success, and they were thrilled to be part of it. They all became our ambassadors in the community.

The hospital picked up steam, and the census grew. We had initially opened one unit of the hospital. When the time came to open the second unit, I needed help. One day I received a call from Steve Heisler, one of my psychiatric residents at Oak Knoll a few years earlier. He said he was completing his Navy obligation in Boston and wondered if there were any opportunities for him at Walnut Creek Hospital. "Get on the next plane," I answered. He did, and we met the next day. We subsequently became life long partners. In our becoming partners we had inadvertently joined the world of group medical practice. In a few months Steve became the Assistant Medical Director and the administrator-teacher of one of the two units of the hospital. We both ran the hospital from a clinical and a marketing point of view, and we thought we learned all of the ins and outs of the psychiatric hospital business.

The use of an ever increasing number of psychiatric drugs plus an enlightened approach to using a psychiatric hospital made the prospects for improvement or cure better than ever before. Optimal care for very sick psychiatric patients was now possible, and we took pride in our newly developed abilities to treat the sickest of the sick.

Some voices were worse than others. "You cunt! You smell! Do it now! You smell of shit!" the voices screamed. They never stopped. This was the worst they had ever been.

Darlene was 20, and this was the third time she had been floridly psychotic since she was age 15. She had not told her parents about the first episode. But the voices were much softer then. She had feigned physical illness to avoid school or seeing her friends. After a few weeks the voices subsided, and she forgot about them.

The second episode, at age 19, was worse. The voices were louder and more frequent. They forcefully commanded her to do certain things as the price for their promised disappearance. But slamming doors or throwing things did not give her the relief the voices had promised. Diagnosed as suffering from schizophrenia, she was hospitalized;

and over a period of a few weeks a new antipsychotic drug, Prolixin, helped her improve. After she
left the hospital, she felt good except for some of
the side effects of the medicine such as muscle
stiffness or involuntary foot tapping. She soon
stopped the medication and did not keep follow-
up appointments with her psychiatrist, an unfortunate mistake.

The latest episode began a few weeks after she
got married. She awoke in the middle of the night
screaming that she wanted to be dead. She told
her husband about the loud voices shouting and
screaming in her head. She then attempted to hit
her head against the wall to make the voices go
away.

She was brought to the hospital and admitted to the high security locked unit. She was soft
spoken and smiled inappropriately as she described her nonstop nightmare. A few minutes
after the admission interview, she raced the length
of the hospital corridor and slammed her head into
the locked fire door at the far end. She knocked
herself unconscious. She was quickly taken to the
emergency room of the general hospital next
door for a head injury evaluation. Fortunately
none was found, and she was returned to Walnut
Creek Hospital.

This time she was restrained to her bed because
she was such a high suicide risk. Soft leather

restraints were applied to both of her arms and to both feet. Since Prolixin had helped her before, she was started on the same medication. At daily staff meetings and at change of shift meetings, all staff members were alerted to the fact that she was a high suicide risk even in the hospital setting. Her restraints were only to be removed for eating or toileting. Eating utensils were to be plastic. We required the staff to repeatedly evaluate Darlene's psychotic symptoms and her suicide potential. Interactions with the staff were all to be on the same theme. All staff reassured her that the voices were not real, that they only seemed real, that they were symptoms of her mental illness, and that with proper treatment the voices would go away. We told her again and again that there was hope for her and that she would feel better.

Darlene was one of those patients who make you think about her a lot. I knew that she would kill herself if we made some thoughtless mistake either in the treatment planning or in its day to day execution by the staff.

As days went by, she did not seem to improve. I became more worried, but not less resolute. There had to be some medication or combination of medications that would help her. I tried raising the dosage of her Prolixin to mega levels, a procedure that had been shown to be effective in the treatment of some other severely ill patients. When

I gave permission for her to walk in the corridor without restraints, she made another attempt to run head long into the locked fire door. This time a watchful staff member intervened and prevented her from injuring herself. I decided that for further walks in the corridor she would have to have her arms restrained to her sides. That would prevent her from accelerating if she made another dash down the corridor in response to her commanding voices.

New regimens of medication were tried. Ultimately a combination of Proketazine and Thorazine seemed to help her. Darlene's hallu-cinations became softer and less frequent. Their content was still the same—always insulting and frequently commanding. She improved to the point where she was attended to the hospital caf-eteria for meals. But her improvement was erratic with occasional setbacks. For instance, one day she stabbed her arm with a metal fork in response to the commands of the voices.

Over several months her hallucinatory voices slowly diminished in volume and frequency. As she improved, she was given more privileges to spend time off the locked unit accompanied by staff. Later she was transferred to the unlocked unit and ultimately discharged. It took about four months for Darlene to recover to the degree that she could safely leave the hospital. This time after discharge she continued to take her medication, and she did keep follow-up psychiatric appointments. The voices completely stopped.

After her psychotic symptoms disappeared, she became able to talk to me about how getting married had been a declaration of independence from her controlling parents. Her guilt about seeking her independence had something to do with precipitating her psychotic episode.

It seemed like a miracle to me and the staff that Darlene survived and made major steps toward recovery. The staff confidence in their work rose to new levels, and they began to believe we could cure anyone.

By 1981 Walnut Creek Hospital was brimming with patients. There was always a waiting list for beds. And as one patient left the hospital, another candidate for admission on the list was notified that the bed would be held for four hours. If the notified patient did not arrive within four hours, the next prospective patient on the waiting list was called. Because of our high occupancy rate I began to talk with Jim Conte about enlarging the hospital.

Conte sent us a string of neophyte hospital administrators in hope that they would learn the secrets of our success and emulate that success at other CPC hospitals. One of those young administrators, Phil Donahue, an energetic well organized ex-marine, took great delight in phoning the corporate home office to announce that the previous month Walnut Creek Hospital had had a census of 103% of capacity. "No," he laughingly insisted, "two patients were not occupying the same bed."

The rapidly spreading reputation of the hospital brought some unusual referrals.

Beaming from ear to ear, Phil raced into my office as soon as he hung up the phone. He almost shouted, "The Shah of _____ is sending us one his generals for treatment." "You're kidding," I replied. But he wasn't.

Treating the General, whose real name I never knew, posed unique problems. I was told he did not speak a word of English; and he traveled with a non-detachable aide who also served as a translator and bodyguard. Because of security concerns he required a large private room on the locked unit from which he and his aide did not emerge throughout his one month long hospitalization. He was to have no contact with other patients and only designated nursing staff were permitted to dispense his medication and to bring meals into his room. Two strange men, whose existence was never acknowledged, were often seen either on foot or in a car near the periphery of the hospital grounds. I assumed these men were part of the General's security force.

The General suffered from heroin addiction. His withdrawal and initial efforts at rehabilitation went well. Each day when I entered his room, he and his aide both sprang to their feet in a posture of ram rod attention and saluted me. I felt embarrassed. After a few days I protested, "General, in this hospital you do not have to jump to your feet when I enter the room." His response, in very clear English, "Doctor, in this hospital you are my General."

After his month of treatment, he returned to his native country where a revolution a few months later led to his imprisonment and execution.

Audrey was twenty-two but appeared to be fourteen. She weighed eighty-four pounds. Her eyes were sunken and devoid of life. Her face was blank. When she spoke, her voice was almost inaudible, her tone a flat monotone. Her pulse and blood pressure were both low, but she was not in shock. I could barely look at her. When I did look, what I saw was a skeleton barely covered by parchment-like skin. I could not see a single muscle.

Her parents presented what for the most part was a commonplace anorexic history. At fourteen she had become weight conscious and figure conscious. She had begun to diet and to exercise rigorously—often more than two hours daily. One evening her mother discovered her in the act of self-induced vomiting. She confessed to her mother that she needed to purge to avoid weight gain, and she rationalized that many of her peers did the same. When she looked in the mirror, even at less than one hundred pounds, she saw herself as obese.

Over the years she'd had periods of treatment by her family physician, a psychiatrist, several counselors, and a dietician. She had been given a number of diets, vitamins, hormones and several antidepressants. She agreed to restrict her exercise but then exercised in secret. In her nonstop efforts to remain thin, she began to use laxatives on a habitual basis. Her condition had waxed and waned, but she was never symptom free. She always felt fat and saw herself as a blimp. Even when she controlled her stuffing and vomiting, she still obsessed about food. She managed to complete high school, but could never hold a job. She continued to live with her parents. Her social life atrophied, and she lived an isolated existence preoccupied with eating, purging, and weight control.

The episode leading to hospitalization developed over several months. Her parents were dimly aware that she was thinner than she'd ever been. When she fainted, her parents called an ambulance, and she was hospitalized at a nearby general hospital. Her electrolyte levels were abnormal, but were corrected over the next twenty-four hours by intravenous fluids. Except for a low pulse rate, her cardiogram was almost normal. All other blood chemistries and hormone levels were commensurate with the pattern expected in someone starving to death. Efforts to encourage her to eat anything met with almost no success. Even though she was physically weak, she fought any attempts to feed her by nasogastric tube. She repeatedly pulled out the tube. In a last ditch effort to save her life, her internist and I agreed that she be transferred to Walnut Creek Hospital.

At the time she was admitted to Walnut Creek, Audrey was oriented to the month and to the year. She did not know the date or the day of the week. She answered questions slowly and after long pauses—often more than a minute. She was aware that if she continued to avoid eating she would die, but she did not seem to care. She insisted that she was not depressed, and that she had never contemplated suicide. She stated that she really did not care about much of anything except staying thin. That was all she thought about. She did not seem to hallucinate. Her only delusion was that she was still fat.

This was no longer ordinary anorexia. This was the preterminal anorexia nervosa I had read about while I was in medical school but had never seen before in real life. Audrey drifted in a kind of miasmic fog—barely in contact with life.

Her treatment plan included nasogastric tube feedings twice a day while her arms were restrained to the bed. Our nursing director, Beverly Collins, gave the nursing staff a refresher course on the placement and management of nasogastric tubes. I did the first tube insertion myself, both to demonstrate to the staff exactly how I wanted it done and to be certain that Audrey had no anatomical blockages that would interfere with proper tube placement. All medication was to be given by nasogastric tube. To avoid secret purging, the nursing staff even accompanied Audrey when she went to the bathroom.

Electrolyte values were to be done on a daily basis. Cardiograms were repeated every three days. Pulse and blood pressure were monitored four times a day. Her internist visited almost daily.

She was restricted to a private room on the locked unit of the hospital. Staff contacts were frequent. The staff saw to it that Audrey was showered and dressed every day. They talked with her about her weight, eating, vomiting, use of laxatives, her distorted body image, her illness, and the gravity of her condition. These issues and her treatment plan were discussed repeatedly in a very matter of fact way. She was weighed daily. She was given occupational therapy projects such as jigsaw puzzles and crossword puzzles. Some of her art therapy projects included drawings of herself as she perceived herself to be. She invariably saw herself as a whale.

We tried to make it clear that her poor nutrition was a life and death issue. Even if she did not care about it now, at some point she would feel better, and it would all matter to her. Until that time came, we would have to take over the motivation for her being alive.

Her medications included an antidepressant, Tofranil, and an antipsychotic medication, Stelazine. (SSRI antidepressants and atypical antipsychotic medications, useful as appetite stimulants, had not yet been developed.) Her regimen of medication and her medication dosages were revised frequently as a result of whether her condition changed or failed to change.

Audrey hated being tube fed. She objected less to the physical discomfort than to the feeling that she was totally helpless as she was being "fattened up." When I told that she would no longer be tube fed if she reached ninety-two pounds for three consecutive days, she attempted to load up on water before her daily weighings.

Within two weeks I knew that the short term battle was won. There would be no code blue procedure to defibrillate Audrey after a cardiac arrest or some other severe arrhythmia. She still looked painfully thin, but the aura of death was no longer in her room.

Fighting the war for her further improvement was a different matter. She was no longer restricted to her room. She agreed to try milk shakes and other nourishing drinks. Lab work was performed less often. Pulse and blood pressure were now measured only once a day. But the staff watched her closely, especially for evidence of exercising or vomiting.

At ninety-two pounds Audrey's feeding tube was removed. She understood and feared that any weight below ninety pounds would result in the resumption of tube feeding. The hospital dietician met with her repeatedly to develop a diet with her input and acceptance, a diet that hopefully she could live with once she got out of the hospital. Attended privileges off the closed unit along with a monitored and restricted exercise program were contingent upon further weight gain. At one hundred pounds, she was transferred to the unlocked unit of the hospital. Her therapy changed to focus on education for proper nutrition and a well defined but restricted exercise program. More attention was paid to helping her develop her social skills thorough interactions with other patients as well as the staff.

After several months Audry was in condition for discharge. By the time she was discharged, she looked radically different. At one hundred four pounds she still looked thin but no longer skeletal. She had some visible muscles in her arms and legs. There was spirit in her voice. She was more aware of life. She had helped develop a diet she thought she could live with. While she still felt she was a lot fatter than she wanted to be, she was less obsessed about eating and weight. She planned to take some junior college courses and was flirting with the idea of becoming a dietician.

Everything seemed to be coming together. I was having fun. The charter doctors had decided that they didn't really like doing the work that hospital practice required, and we rarely saw them.The medical staff now consisted of a group of very skilled energetic clinicians who fit well into our hospital model. The department heads and the rest of the staff developed pride in our clinical achievements. This was all the result of our increasing ability to help most of the sickest patients to improve. Every difficult patient presented a challenge that we believed we could meet.

Our biggest problems were now elsewhere.

XVI. EMERGENCE OF THE MEDICAL EVILDOERS

As our arsenal of psychiatric drugs grew and our skills in using them increased, by the 1980s anyone with a mental illness stood an excellent chance of symptom relief or at least control of the illness to the point where it was less disabling. By the 1990s the ambitious albeit somewhat unrealistic goal of cure was becoming more openly discussed in professional circles. For the first time in history, the enemy to excellent care in psychiatry was no longer mental illness itself. The science required for success in treatment was now in place, and treatment techniques were being refined. At long last a majority of mentally ill patients could be successfully treated within a reasonable period of time.

But it was too soon to celebrate. Major enemies to optimal treatment were still present. The new enemies were government bureaucrats and the insurance industry.

In 1980 the hospital business was exciting. New hospitals were being built to replace old obsolete hospitals or to meet the needs of a growing population. In one of its never ending but badly flawed attempts at holding down healthcare costs, the Federal government had legislated that a difficult to obtain Certificate of Need should be required to build any new hospital or to add beds to existing hospitals. They reasoned that if new hospital beds existed, hospitals would fill all of the available beds through liberal admission policies or to employ new healthcare technologies. According to the bureaucrats, patients who did not really need hospital care somehow would be enticed to enter hospitals if beds were available. They reasoned that if there were fewer hospital beds that could be filled with sick patients, hospital revenues and healthcare costs thereby would be held in check. They wishfully stated that the actual medical need for the beds would magically disappear. Was this crazy thinking? Of course!

The upshot was easily predictable. To almost no one's surprise, people still became very ill, and the need for hospital beds did not go away. Waiting lists for admission to hospitals became commonplace. The pressure to discharge patients prematurely, once characteristic of only the county hospitals, now spread across the whole system of care.

The Certificate of Need (CON) laws effectively granted monopolies to entities that owned existing hospital beds. Under the law, new Certificate of Need boards were politically appointed to consider, and usually to deny, any proposed expansion of hospital bed capacity. Existing bed owners were almost guaranteed that no new competitor would be permitted to come into what they envisioned were their territories. Assured that their beds would always be filled to near capacity, the value of their existing beds multiplied. With the increase in value of each bed, the hospital companies hired bands of lobbyists to besiege the CON boards to protect or promote their interests.

Despite the CON law, the bureaucrats, and the efforts of stake holder lobbyists to maintain the status quo, some increase in the number of psychiatric beds was possible. But it was a struggle. At Walnut Creek Hospital we obtained several CONs during two expansion phases. The hospital was enlarged from sixty-six beds to eighty-six and later to one hundred twenty beds.

When we applied to the CON boards for permission to expand, according to the rules of the game we were forbidden to contact CON board members directly. All formal contact with the CON board was through an unsupportive, usually openly hostile CON staff. They recognized that their mission was to limit the number of hospital beds, and that their very jobs depended on it. Their recommendations to the board were invariably negative, usually supported by bogus formulas and bogus statistics which we were certain they made up as they went along. To be successful in our efforts to gain CON board approval, we had to somehow or other to bypass the negative CON staff.

To gain access to the board and provide them with information other than the distorted reports of the CON staff, we contacted friends and associates of board members, family members, employers, politicians—anyone with possible access. And we made our pitch for more beds. My partner, Steve Heisler, now the assistant medical director, was very talented at spreading our message through influential circles. By the time of the public meetings of the CON board we knew almost how many positive votes we had, and how many votes were going to go against us.

The bureaucratic staff of the CON board always argued that according to some arcane formula, which had nothing to do with reality, there were already more than enough psychiatric beds in our area to meet patients' needs for decades to come. They made the same argument no matter how many patients in real life were being denied access to care because there were not enough hospital beds to take care of them. After awhile even the CON boards became skeptical of their own staff's boiler-plate arguments.

While the outcome of a CON board meeting was largely predetermined, board meetings were always dramatic events enacted before large audiences in crowded rooms. Lobbyists would testify that only the existing facilities they represented could do an adequate job of meeting the community's mental health needs. Neighbors would argue that more beds might be needed, but only if they were built in neighborhoods other than theirs. Civil rights groups would decry the existence of psychiatric hospitals altogether and urged that all psychiatric hospitals be closed down. Satisfied former patients recounted how their optimal treatment had saved or radically changed their lives.

Sometimes even patients with the most severe problems realized that they needed help. Fred looked like the killer in anyone's nightmare. All of his life he had struggled with the urge to kill people. He joined the marines as an outlet for his homicidal cravings and was proud of a large number of "registered kills" while he was a sniper in Vietnam. Back in civilian life, as an outlet for his urges to kill people, he lured muggers to assault him first so that he could hurt them with some sense of justification.When he recognized his urges were getting even more out of control, he sought treatment at Walnut Creek Hospital. At the time of his admission, he explained that he did not want to murder innocent strangers.

Two years after his period of successful treatment at the hospital, to our amazement Fred appeared at a CON board meeting where we were applying for additional beds. Because of his appearance and demeanor, he radiated an aura of power and barely controlled evil. His very presence brought the CON board to silent fear-ful attention. To their surprise he argued that the hospital needed more beds to keep people like him from wandering around the streets. He was absolutely right, and the board, transcending the negative staff recommendations, accepted our proposal to expand the hospital.

After a decade the CON laws were repealed. An ini-tial frantic burst of hospital building slowed significantly as the marketplace laws of supply and demand plus our increased ability to use out patient services more effectively limited the need for new hospital construc-tion. Psychiatrists' ability to treat more patients in out of hospital settings greatly increased as a result of the intro-duction and use of new antipsychotic, antianxiety and antidepressant medications.

Insurance carriers have always been confused about psychiatric care. With the advent of psychiatric drugs and the possibility of improvement and cure, insurance covering psychiatric hospital care became possible. The problem was that the insurance carriers did not under-stand the need for psychiatric hospital treatment—even emergency life saving care. They often refused to pay for the very services they had promised to provide to their plan members. Weeks after discharge, patients and their families might receive a denial of payment letter for claims covering their psychiatric hospital care. The rationale for the denial of payment rarely made good sense, if any sense at all, and we encouraged patients to appeal to the insurance companies, county medical societies, and their congressmen or, if necessary, to take legal action. We wrote reports or even went to court to support their claims. Somehow with continuing effort our patients were almost always successful in their attempts to force their insurance carriers to pay for their hospital care. Blue Cross was so confused that it ultimately sent an executive vice president to visit us at Walnut Creek Hospital to examine what was happening. At the end of a full day he stated that he had learned a lot, and he had concluded that what we were doing was clinically correct and justifiable. Seeing us as pioneers he jokingly added, "You can always identify a pioneer by the number of arrows he has sticking out of his ass." I considered his comment a disquieting compliment.

But the result of his visit was disappointing. There was no enlightened change in the troubled relationship between the insurance carrier and the hospital. We were the pioneers, and the arrows kept flying. Blue Cross then hired a psychiatrist who, based on his review of patients' medical records, made a series of clinical judgments that the inpatient psychiatric care we provided was almost never a medical necessity. His pronouncements led to a plethora of denials of payment for care that had already been provided. I contacted him to help me understand the rationale for his judgments. He explained his view that no patient who was on the unlocked unit of the hospital really needed hospital care in the first place, and that anyone on the locked unit should be treated on the open unit. When I challenged his expertise, he confessed that he had very little experience treating patients who required psychiatric hospital care.

Frustrated at his response, we took a new tack. We contacted the staff of Sixty Minutes. They expressed interest in doing a TV program on insurance company fraud. When they contacted Blue Cross to try to set up a meeting with the CEO, the insurance company refused to reply. The next week the Blue Cross reviewing psychiatrist was terminated.

Fighting with insurance carriers on a case by case basis was a nuisance and very time consuming. Denial of payment frightened patients and their families who now saw themselves facing bills they were usually unable to pay. But as a result of our determination to fight every denial and our track record of ultimate success in those fights, the insurance carriers, including Blue Cross, largely backed off. At least for treatment at Walnut Creek Hospital, they stopped denying payment for in patient psychiatric care.

Elsewhere, however, the insurance carriers did not back off. At various medical meetings other psychiatric hospital medical directors told me one story after another of inappropriate denials of payment for care.

Then the insurance carriers made a move that changed the whole character of delivery of health care in the United States. It started in California. All it took was a few small, almost invisible changes in the state Welfare and Institutions Code. Prior to these few changes, the W&I Code had mandated that patients were to have a universe of choice in selecting clinicians and hospitals. To usher in the era of managed care took only the insertion of the word "not" in a few key sections of the code. Heavily promoted by the insurance carrier lobbyists, legislation was introduced which in essence amends a statement such as, "Patients shall be entitled to a universe of choice of providers" to "Patients shall not be entitled to a universe of choice of providers." The enacting bill sailed through the legislature with the majority of legislators having no understanding whatever of the potential consequences of passage. The governor had some warning. He didn't sign the bill, but he didn't veto the bill, either. Within thirty days the legislature-approved but unsigned bill became law.

The full force of the legislation struck me the day after it had been passed by the legislature. When I read about it in the morning paper, I wanted to scream and punch holes in the walls. I was horrified at the prospects for the future. As a result of these key changes in the law, insurance carriers suddenly would have all of the power to determine health care. If patients no longer had access to all doctors or hospitals, they could be ordered to receive care only from those providers with whom the insurance carrier had a contract. The insurance carriers now could push doctors and hospitals around by the threat of not contracting with them. Without contracts with the insurance carriers, the clinicians and hospitals would be denied the ability to provide service to huge pools of insured patients who might need treatment. Even if they did have a contract to provide care, doctors and hospitals under the new contracting process between providers and insurance carriers, the insurance carriers were empowered to set rates for care. With the threat of excluding specific providers from their approved lists, the insurance companies began the process of lowering rates they paid to doctors and to hospitals. Without contracts with the insurance carriers or even with contracts at new very low rates, some providers could be driven out of business.

"What makes you think you have the God given right to exist?" The outgoing president of Blue Cross of Southern California was angrily addressing a very large group of hospital administrators and CEOs a few weeks after the blockbuster managed care legislation care had became law in California.

Whether we said it or not, most of us did believe that we were doing God's work in facilitating the treatment of sick people in well-run hospitals. We sincerely believed that hospitals were necessary places where people could receive treatment and get well. Now here was this demon from hell threatening us with the prospect of closing some of our hospitals and stopping us from fulfilling our mission. And we were cowering before him because we realized that, armed with the changed Welfare and Institutions Code, he might really have the power to do what he was threatening to do.

This devil from Blue Cross now represented the entire insurance industry. Their lobbying with members of the California State legislature had led to the passage of this landmark piece of managed care legislation. The power to determine hospital care had now shifted from patients and their doctors to uncaring insurance carriers. Once it began in California, insurance carriers were successful in promoting similar legislation in the other states.

I was frantic. I tried to present my understanding of the problem to the governing counsel of the Northern California Psychiatric Society. I even had a plan for the Society to contract with the insurance carriers to review quality of care in order to protect patient treatment under the new laws. The Psychiatric Society counsel thought I was crazy. At that time they did not understand what was happening. They wanted to pretend the problem didn't exist. Later when reality forced them to understand, their fear was so great that they were paralyzed to act. In retrospect, it was probably too late anyway. Organized psychiatry, even if it had been able to face reality, was quite helpless to stem the tide that was to result in the limitations managed care imposed on optimal psychiatric treatment.

The impact on psychiatric hospital care was major. Insurance companies now assigned so-called case managers to individual patients. The case managers' skill lay in badgering hospitals and individual clinicians to limit lengths of stay by posing pseudo clinical arguments. Their explicit threat was always denial of payment. Evne when care was approved, the approval came in one or two day portions after more time consuming phone calls from attending doctors being required to extend the duration of hospital care. Most clinicians did not want to spend time on the phone each day fighting with bogus case managers. Rather than argue, they often acceded to the case managers' demands to limit hospital care.

Here is part of an actual telephone conversation between a psychiatrist and a case manager.

Doctor: "George is 47 and has lost his job. He is very depressed, and he now believes his family would be better off if he were dead. He has made two suicide attempts before, and he is suicidal now. He needs psychiatric hospitalization to avert a catastrophe."

Case Manager: "What makes you think he is suicidal now?"

Dr: "He wants to be dead. He is not able to sleep. He feels worthless. He is irritable. He is withdrawn. He is eating poorly and has lost fifteen pounds in the last month. He is obsessing about different ways of killing himself."

CM: "Does he have a specific plan?"

Dr: "He thinks about hanging himself or sitting in his car in the garage with the motor running."

CM: "Has he actually tried to harm himself?"

Dr: "Well, no. Not this time."

CM: "When did he make his previous suicide attempts?"

Dr: "About four or five years ago. He took an over-dose of pills both times, and he was hospitalized."

CM: "So nothing recent?"

Dr: "No. But so what? He is actively suicidal now."

CM: "How long has he been thinking of suicide?"

Dr: "I'm not sure. I think it has been the last few weeks. But the urge is stronger now."

CM: "And he hasn't tried to harm himself?"

Dr: "Does he actually have to make a suicide attempt to merit getting into a hospital that will protect him?"

CM: "How about intensive outpatient care? We can assign him a therapist who will see him several times a week. You can continue to manage his medication on an outpatient basis."

Dr: "You don't get it. If this man is not put into a protective environment today, he may end up dead. This is serious!"

CM: " I can authorize intensive out patient care. But it doesn't sound like inpatient care is indicated."

Dr: "What is your skill level?"

CM: "I have a master's degree in psychology."

Dr: "Have you experience in working with severely ill patients?"

CM: "No. But I have certain guidelines that we follow."

Dr: "You are not going to authorize life saving hospital care for someone who is on the verge of a serious suicide attempt?"

CM: "I did not say he couldn't go into a hospital. I said that according to our guidelines, we won't pay for his hospital care."

Dr: "Can I speak to a psychiatrist?"

CM: "I will refer this case for medical review."

Dr: "Will a psychiatrist review the case and call me back?"

CM: "A doctor, not necessarily a psychiatrist, or a Ph.D. psychologist will review the case. You will receive a decision in one or two working days." (Click)

The psychiatrist admitted George to the hospital for life saving protection and intensive treatment. The insurance carrier initially denied payment for George's hospital care but later, after a lengthy appeal process, reversed the decision.

Hospitals came to fear the retroactive denial of payment by insurance carriers and the time consuming and costly appeal processes necessary to receive payment. And to make matters worse, their appeals were not always successful. The hospitals, to avoid loss from the retrospective denial of claims by insurance carriers, took to hiring their own utilization review nurses. Their job was to harass the attending physicians into premature patient discharge. In efforts to assuage the insurance carrier case managers, the utilization review nurses often became more tyrannical than the insurance company case managers themselves. The treating physicians would then have to fight with the hospital utilization review nurses to see that their patients received the hospital care they actually needed.

Many doctors grew tired of this extra burden and came to acquiesce to the utilization review nurse's judgments. Some even retired prematurely. Others opted to stop treating patients in hospitals. Instead of referring patients for hospital care, physicians would send patients to emergency rooms and hope for the best.

Hospital care in most hospitals is now left to a group of doctors called 'hospitalists'. Their work is almost exclusively the care of hospitalized patients. Because their work is quite specialized, they are quite skilled and usually do a very good job. But lengths of stay are more often determined by the utilization review nurses than the physicians' professional judgments.

For now, the insurance carriers have won control of the health care treatment system. Under the guise of managed care they have gained the ability to control many major treatment decisions. Just to get a diagnostic procedure or surgical procedure done on a non-emergency basis may require weeks of delay to obtain an insurance carrier preauthorization. Unless their doctors are able and willing to put up a good fight, all too often patients are deprived of the care they thought they were insured to receive.

Hospital stays for psychiatric patients are shorter by far. Optimal psychiatric inpatient care is now history. Many patients who are seriously ill are denied hospital admission altogether. Of those admitted, most are discharged prematurely; often long before they are really ready to manage their lives in the world outside of the hospital. A compromise between the hospitals and insurance carriers has been the development of less expensive partial hospital programs where patients, discharged after a few days of hospital care, live at home and appear at the hospital for a treatment program five days a week.

Until the last few years psychiatric patients have continued to be the victims of insurance carrier discrimination. Many insurers had placed severe, often unrealistic restrictions on how much care mental health patients could receive. For a good number of insurance contracts outpatient psychiatric care was limited to twenty visits per year, or inpatient care was restricted to thirty days in any given year. These restrictions on the amount of care provided for mental health patients have negatively impacted patients' treatment.

It has taken more than a decade for congressional intervention and additional legislation to partially tame managed care company avarice and uncaring behavior. Many states and finally the federal government have now passed bills demanding 'parity', mandating that insurance carriers provide coverage for mentally ill patients the same way that they provide care for patients with medical or surgical problems. Under this 'parity' legislation those patients with diagnoses such as major depression, bipolar illness, or schizophrenia, gain access to the amount of psychiatric care necessary for the treatment of their illnesses; the amount of care may not be arbitrarily restricted.

Nonetheless for patients with serious psychiatric illness the hospital revolving door, once restricted to the county hospital systems, is now almost the rule. Under Obamacare the rationing of mental health care resources is almost a certainty. And the quality of care will suffer, not because an optimal level of care does not exist, but because it will be denied by government bureaucrats who will act with far less concern for quality of care than even the private insurance carriers. Complaints and appeals to insurance companies often pay off. Complaints to government run agencies most often lead to a frustrating run around that makes the private insurance carriers look benign and generous.

XVII. THE HEALING MACHINE

"Are there any more bids?" The auctioneer paused as he looked around the crowded room. "Going once! Going twice! Going three times! Sold to East Bay Hospital Corporation!"

The scene was not an auction house. It was a bankruptcy court in 1982. The presiding judge had turned the proceedings over to Charles Duck, the bankruptcy trustee for the defunct Richmond Hospital. Duck had conducted the auction in the courtroom with three bidders punching up the price in the presence of a happy almost cheering gaggle of creditors, all envisioning a big payoff. After the auction was over, the judge approved the sale. The bank was to be paid off in full. The creditors received most of what they claimed was due to them. And East Bay Hospital Corporation ended up with the remaining assets of Richmond Hospital. Later I read somewhere that Duck had embezzled some of the proceeds and was imprisoned.

Steve Heisler and I were present in the courtroom along with Mike Richardson, representing our investment banking firm of Birr Wilson, and our corporate attorney, Phil Boesche. Steve and I were the major shareholders of Psychiatric Health Services which in turn owned all of the shares of East Bay Hospital Corporation. The other bidders included the Wahl Medical Group, which wanted to convert the remains of Richmond Hospital into an outpatient surgical clinic to complement the two other surgical clinics they already owned and operated. The third bidder was a mysterious woman who made only one bid during the course of the auction.

A major difference between us and the Wahl Group was that we didn't have any money. The Wahl Group attorney caught everyone's attention in the court room by waving a cashier's check for one million dollars. The message of the gesture was to indicate that they had real money. In comparison we had only the presence and the promise of our investment banking firm that we would raise whatever money was required. This difference in substance between the bidders was not lost upon the trustee. He asked the judge to accept a $600,000 differential in bids between bidders with real money and those without any money. That meant that to exceed the Wahl Group opening bid of one million dollars cash, we had to bid more than one million six hundred thousand dollars.

Neither Steve nor I had ever been in a situation even remotely like this before. It all felt like a bizarre dream. We were both scared. After all, we were doctors. We treated patients. We didn't know anything about this strange world of mega dollars. Did we really want to do this? We then looked at our investment banker who smiled a shark-like smile and told us to go ahead. I looked over to Steve to be certain that he understood Richardson's advice. Steve said something like, "Go for it."

I put up my hand and bid one million six hundred fifty thousand dollars. I discovered a giddy feeling that comes from just being able to say numbers that big and to be taken seriously. While it didn't feel real to me, I was happy to play this fantasy game. More anxious and euphoric bidding followed. In difficult years afterward, only half in jest Steve often said that we had lost the auction as we ended up owning the hospital.

Had Jim Conte of Community Psychiatric Centers been less arrogant a year earlier, none of this would have happened. Steve and I would have continued to work at Walnut Creek Hospital, enjoying our performance based bonus derived from the hospital's record profits. Conte had other ideas. While he was unilaterally abrogating my profit sharing contractual arrangement with CPC, he had said, "Harv, you are already the best paid part time medical director in the country. How can you afford to give it up?" My protests reminding him of our long-standing profit-sharing agreement went for naught. Shortly afterward I heard through others in the company that Conte had boasted about how he was now limiting my salary, that he could "cut off any doctor's balls."

I had always known that Conte was a man who could not be trusted. My awareness had been underscored by what we all knew was his recent betrayal of the brightest, most talented and most ambitious of his executives. John Hughes had been a high powered yet sensitive young man whose brilliance and integrity radiated from across the room. It was Hughes who had been responsible for expanding the number of CPC hospitals in the United States and more recently the opening of CPC hospitals in the UK (despite the government run health system). It was a shock to all of us that Hughes had left the company after Conte had broken their incentivised agreement. Within a few years Hughes opened his own company in the UK, Cygnet Health Care, and began to enjoy wonderful success as he built his company into a dominant player in UK health.

So why was I surprised when Conte knifed me? Conte's refusal to perform under the terms of my contract left me feeling hurt and betrayed, at first, and then depressed. But after a few weeks, my hurt and depression turned to anger and scheming. Steve and I began planning for our own company. If Hughes could do it, so could we. My trust in Steve and my faith in our ability to work together had become very strong. He in turn had confidence that we would be successful no matter what we opted to do. Our track record to date at Walnut

Creek Hospital was undeniable proof that we had the skills and talents to be winners in the hospital business.

In a way Steve and I really did know a lot about how to run a psychiatric hospital. We knew how to develop great treatment delivery systems that produced results. Equally important we knew how to market those systems. But we were very weak on the business end, even though I had learned a fair amount during our years at Walnut Creek Hospital. Even running a medical practice was easy compared to running a hospital. Steve and I knew just enough to know that there was a lot we did not know. We needed a hotshot hospital administrator to join us.

Early in our planning for the new business we sadly concluded that we could not compete in the hospital industry. Companies with billions of dollars were stalking the country like Tyrannosaurus Rex devouring existing hospitals and buying off Certificate of Need boards to get permission for monopolistic growth. We had almost no money to invest in our business, and we were uncertain that we would be able to raise enough capital to get started. It felt as though we didn't have a chance to become a player in the industry.

An alternative niche might be a health resort that featured counseling and fitness. Our program would provide diet supervision and health education. At the time the concept was somewhat novel, and we were afraid that the idea might not catch on. The mental health oriented health spa concept seemed too flaky and too uncertain, and after awhile we gave up on it.We felt far more knowledgeable and more comfortable in operating psychiatric hospitals.Therefore we opted to move on into the psychiatric hospital business, even if it were a territory inhabited by man eating corporate monsters.

We hired someone to scout out hospital acquisition opportunities. But we didn't know how to pick a development person, and we chose the wrong person for the job. Within a few months we decided to do our own development. At the same time we took on a new partner who was designated to become our hotshot administrator. Richard Ponder was the successful and ambitious administrator of a large general hospital in Las Vegas. He had been having serious problems on his very active psychiatric in-patient service. On hearing of my success at Walnut Creek Hospital, Ponder had invited me to act as a consultant to help straighten things out. I flew to Las Vegas to review his psychiatric operations. It wasn't difficult to identify the key problems and formulate some reasonable solutions. Ponder liked my analysis and the plan I proposed. We got on well. During the few days we worked together, we developed mutual respect. A few weeks later Steve and I invited Ponder to join us in our proposed psychiatric hospital business. Ponder was interested in becoming a principal in a start-up company, and we worked out the details of his involvement as a prospective shareholder. Ponder was slated to become the administrator of whatever hospital we were ultimately to acquire. But it was to be up to me and Steve to identify and somehow acquire the first hospital in what we fantasized would be our own hospital chain.

We then heard that French Hospital in San Francisco had failed in its attempt to run a chemical dependency unit, and it had been closed down. Emphasizing our success at Walnut Creek Hospital, Steve and I pitched a management contract proposal to the French Hospital board of directors. We claimed that we would resurrect their failed chemical dependency program, make it successful, and ultimately convert it into an even more successful acute psychiatric inpatient service. The costs to French would be far lower than those they had incurred in their failed program under a contract with a nationally known chemical dependency management company. Our costs would be low too. So would our potential profits. But even more important for us, the project would launch our company into the hospital industry world. Once you are a real player, people take you seriously. We could then make acquisition bids that others would find credible. We could more easily obtain government permits. Most important, we could raise money. The disadvantages in our French Hospital management contract were that our upside potential was limited, and that French had the option of canceling the contract at the end of each year.

After the French Hospital board came to tour always bustling Walnut Creek Hospital, they accepted our proposal. Steve Heisler and I then established a corporate

entity, Psychiatric Health Services, under which to conduct our new business. Word spreads quickly in the hospital world, and I soon received a call from Jim Conte.
Always suspicious of any conceivable threat to his
own business, he asked what we were doing at French
Hospital, and what was the nature of Psychiatric Health
Services? "Consulting" was my partially true response.
We had not actually restarted the French Hospital drug
and alcohol treatment program at the time. But I would
have happily lied to Conte had there been the need. He
had broken our long-standing agreement about profit
sharing at Walnut Creek Hospital, and I no longer had
any sense of loyalty to him.

Steve and I felt increasingly excited at the prospect
of starting our own business. Soon the French Hospital
management contract was signed, and we really were
in business. At the same time through Palmer Watson,
a far sighted clergyman with a special interest in mental health, we first heard about the shuttered Richmond
Hospital, universally known to be a wreck of the worst
order, a place in total disrepair. Watson urged us to have
a look at the place.

To build a company in the hospital industry Steve and
I knew we had to have money or access to money. We
quickly found that regular banks would have nothing
to do with a start up company like ours. But aggressive
investment banking firms might have interest. The first
few companies we visited barely listened to our presen-
tation. The third company, Birr Wilson, had had a positive

experience with a psychiatric hospital company. Ten years earlier they had underwritten the common stock offering of Community Psychiatric Centers. And the immense success of CPC had become part of their own success story. Because they were familiar with the psychiatric hospital industry, Birr Wilson could easily evaluate the potential of any project that Steve and I proposed. They were impressed that Steve and I operated Walnut Creek Hospital, CPC's most profitable hospital, and that we had signed a management contract with French Hospital. Our role in these two operations convinced them that we were a young but knowledgeable management capable of success in our own venture. One of the firm's founders, Ted Birr, turned us over to Mike Richardson, a very creative and fiercely aggressive underwriter of junk bonds. Our agreement with Birr Wilson was that Steve and I had to come up with a hospital that might be an acquisition candidate, and Birr Wilson would issue and market an Industrial Development Bond.

Richmond Hospital became our prime candidate. The hospital, now closed down, had been a, derelict "bombed out" acute care general hospital located in Richmond, California. It never had had a psychiatric unit. The hospital had originally opened in the 1940s when Richmond was the flourishing home of the World War II naval shipyards. Decades later, a new hospital had been built in the adjacent city of San Pablo. Most of the medical staff and their patients were attracted by the new hospital. Richmond Hospital began to suffer from an antique physical plant, the desertion of much of the medical staff, and a falling patient census. Under a series of inept administrators, already deferred maintenance of the hospital physical plant was deferred even longer, and vital hospital systems for billing and collecting fell apart. The result was closure and bankruptcy.

The wreck of the hospital, its vintage, and what was now an undesirable location left little prospect that it would ever be reopened. Hospital chains whose growth was hampered by CON boards were eager to buy any existing licensed facilities. But after examination of the Richmond Hospital physical plant, the books, and demographics of the area, they all concluded that this particular hospital was a hopeless prospect at any price, and no hospital company came forward with an offer.

For us the beauty of Richmond Hospital was its very ugliness and hopelessness. If no one with real money wanted the hospital, it could be affordable for us.

How ugly was it? Very ugly! The fire marshal counted more than two hundred wall perforations. No major system was intact.What did work was either badly worn or obsolete. The roof was more like a showerhead than an overhead shelter against the elements.

Any other hospital with obvious potential was totally unaffordable. Four months earlier Steve and I had made a bid to acquire a dingy freestanding psychiatric hospital in Whiskey Hill (later renamed Morgan Hill). Our two million-dollar bid seemed to make good business sense to us. But it did not compare to the four and one half million dollars bid by a non profit hospital chain intent on moving into the area and willing to pay a premium to get there.

Our winning bid on Richmond Hospital was two million six hundred thousand dollars. But the Industrial Development bonds we issued a few months later totaled six million dollars. In our prospectus we had made it clear to prospective investors in the bonds that, beyond the purchase price, we needed money for repair and to operate the hospital for more than the first year.

We reopened, with the new name of East Bay Hospital, as an acute care general hospital. We had an emergency room, an intensive care unit, and a labor and delivery unit apart from medical and surgical beds. As much as we wanted to open a psychiatric unit, we couldn't do it. The limitations imposed by the absurd but suffocating Certificate of Need laws made it impossible to reopen the hospital unless we had exactly the same type of beds as had existed in Richmond hospital. To our disappointment when we reopened the hospital after it had been closed for more than a year, the hospital performed poorly. Almost all of the community doctors had now gotten used to using the newer hospital in San Pablo, and very few were interested in returning to East Bay Hospital.

Ponder had many talents as an administrator; but it turned out that cost control was not amongst them. And the hospital was far more expensive to renovate than we had planned. Furthermore, with insufficient revenue coming in to offset the costs, the cost of operation seemed astronomical. It became painfully clear that operating a general hospital was far different than running a psychiatric hospital. I still maintained my psychiatric practice, but more and more of my time was spent before a computer working with spread sheets, charting the future course of East Bay Hospital. And I did not like what the spreadsheets predicted. It was all downhill. Every day I stared at the timetable for the death of our fledgling business.

That first year it felt as though we went out of business thousands of times. I dreaded Wednesday afternoon meetings with Steve Heisler and Dick Ponder. Each time we met we had to face the painful fact that there was not enough money for the hospital to survive. Where could we find the money to make payroll on Fridays? Where was the cash to make our payroll tax payments? How could we deal with creditors such as food vendors, hospital supply, laundry and utilities whose services we absolutely needed to remain open?

My spread sheet analysis told me to face the most miserable truth. We could not possibly survive if we were to continue to operate as a general hospital. Contrary to the opinion of an expensive consulting firm we had hired, I decided that we needed to close the hospital down to stop our drain of cash. We needed to use what cash we still had to remodel part of the hospital as a psychiatric unit. Of course we would have to struggle through the political process of facing a Certificate of

Need Board whose staff foolishly insisted that no new psychiatric beds were needed in our area. In reality there were no psychiatric hospital beds at all in our half of the County. And the CON staff negative opinion would be strongly supported by the hospitals that already had psychiatric units, including Walnut Creek Hospital, which did not want to see any new hospital compete for patients—especially one run by me and Steve. Fortunately, through Steve's special talent for lobbying, we found ourselves with many friends in the community and in the state capital. It was a blatant reality that there were no psychiatric beds in the East Bay Hospital area, and we did prevail in the political process.

When we first reopened the hospital with a wing of psychiatric beds, patients were referred to fill them almost at once. Some of our old medical and professional staff at Walnut Creek Hospital, unhappy with the direction of that hospital after our departure, came to join us at East Bay Hospital. Other psychiatrists, new to the area, came to work with us. Over time we converted more and more beds to psychiatry, and with each addition of beds, patients from all over the San Francisco Bay Area and beyond were referred to fill them. After a few years almost all of our beds were psychiatric beds. At the same time, the hated Certificate of Need laws were repealed.

The hospital at last was a success. Steve and I had known all along how to run a psychiatric hospital. Ponder opted to resign, a casualty of the stress of trying to resurrect East Bay Hospital. We bought back his shares of the company. Next we found a Chief Financial Officer, Sid Lundwall, who was experienced in working through serious financial problems. Lundwall was sufficiently creative to give us viable options that had never occurred to us. Finally we realized that Lois Patsy, our Director of Nursing who had become interim hospital administrator, was a cost conscious capable leader. She became the new administrator.

Our mission as a hospital became clearer. Patients with severe chronic mental illness often became unable to hold jobs. Jobless and with dwindling resources, they fell into the economic class that could only receive healthcare under the Medicaid or Medicare programs. These were usually patients whom free standing psychiatric hospitals both did not want to treat or were unable to admit as a result of laws excluding them from receiving Medicaid payments. They were also patients who, because of the severity of their illness and ugliness of their behavior, acute care general hospitals were unable to treat and usually did not want to treat. These patients were too sick. They were too crazy. They were too messy. They were too suicidal. They were to too combative. They were even homicidal. No one wanted them. The crowded county hospitals, where they usually received short-term help under the revolving door model of care, were unable to provide more than Band-Aid treatment. And emergency rooms throughout the nine county

Bay Area were desperate to have some constructive resource. East Bay Hospital became that resource.

Patients could be admitted to East Bay Hospital at any time of the day or night, whenever the emergent need arose, and were assigned to the psychiatrist on call. A treatment plan was initiated at once. The plan would then be modified from day to day as a function of the patient's improvement or lack thereof. Patients saw psychiatrists seven days a week. Each unit of the hospital had a ward preceptor, a salaried hospital psychiatrist who functioned as an administrator-teacher for the unit. His job was to review each case at a multidisciplinary case conference five mornings per week and to conduct doctors rounds three days a week. The attending psychiatrists all made brief visits to the team meetings to review their patients with the staff and the preceptor. Treatment plans were often fleshed out or modified, and everyone was made clear about what his or her role was to be in each patient's treatment. Everyone on the unit staff was included in each patient's treatment.

It all sounded good, but it still wasn't easy; not for us, and not for the patient.

That man lying next to Janice in bed was the Devil. God had warned her. She carefully sneaked into the kitchen. Armed with her longest and sharpest knife, she quietly stole back to the bedroom. Then she stabbed the man with all of her might. She stabbed him again and again. At last the Devil was dead.

Janice, in a psychotic state, had murdered her husband. She was released from prison after seven years. After her release she refused to see a psychiatrist for follow-up care. Six months later, she stopped taking her antipsychotic drug, Haldol, because she did not like the way it made her feel. She knew the medicine made her drool and feel stiff. Without it her physical symptoms went away. She even felt more alert. But within a few weeks she began to hear God's voice talking to her again. She became sleepless and confused. When police apprehended her for smashing out several car windshields, she screamed that God was sending her to do his work and that she was special.

She was taken to the county hospital emergency room, which in turn sent her to East Bay Hospital. She was bound in leather restraints at the time of her admission. Still in restraints, she was carefully transferred from the hospital gurney to a seclusion room bed. Because of her psychotic and unpredictably violent behavior, the continued use of restraints seemed mandatory for her protection and the safety of all those around her.

Apart from her commanding auditory hallucinations and delusions that others were out to kill her, her thinking jumped from subject to subject at about one sentence intervals. For the most part she was more intent upon listening to and responding to her voices than to the treatment staff.

Frequent staff contacts all focused on helping her to regain her grasp of reality. Her doctor and the hospital staff all told Janice that she was ill and that her voices were symptoms of her illness and not real. Her psychiatrist decided that rather than resume her old medication, he would prescribe a newer antipsychotic, Risperdal, which seemed to have a far lower incidence of unpleasant side effects. He reasoned that patients with serious mental illness would be more likely to keep on taking medications if these drugs had fewer side effects.

Janice improved slowly over a period of a month. As she improved, she was given privileges to participate in other treatment programs at the hospital. She was then transferred to the unlocked unit. During the last ten days of her hospital stay she made good sense when she talked. She became completely free of hallucinations and persecutory delusions. She was able to acknowledge that she had a serious mental illness. She recalled with regret that she had murdered her husband. She had some appreciation of her need for the indefinite use of antipsychotic medications and stated that she much preferred the Risperdal. She was discharged to a board and care home, and arrangements were made for her to see a psychiatrist for continuing outpatient treatment.

In contrast to the homicidal patients, others, like Greg, were highly suicidal.

When he was first seen at the hospital, he confessed, "Shouldn't I be dead?" It was his right to die, and he deserved to die, Greg reasoned. As he saw it, he was a failure in life. Three years earlier he had lost his company and his fortune. He was not certain if his partner had anything to do with it, but he concluded that it was all due to his own bad judgment.

Greg, his wife, and three teen-aged children now lived in reduced circumstances. Two years prior to his being admitted to East Bay Hospital he deliberately drove his car into a tree and lost most of his right leg. He was sorry he had survived. He subsequently made three other suicide attempts, all by an overdose of pills taken after he had had too much to drink. Each time he was hospitalized elsewhere for a few days. He would then insist that he was no longer suicidal, and he would be discharged to outpatient treatment. He had seen several different psychiatrists. They had prescribed a long list of antidepressant medications, none of which seemed to have much beneficial effect. He refused a recommendation that he have electric shock treatment.

He took another serious drug overdose, and this time he required medical care on an intensive care unit. Despite Greg's protests, a consulting psychiatrist insisted on sending him to East Bay Hospital on an involuntary basis.

He was admitted to the locked unit of the hospital. At the time he was admitted, he was well groomed and apparently cheerful. He joked and smiled as he argued that his transfer to East Bay Hospital was only due to the consulting psychiatrist's fear of malpractice liability. He insisted that there was no reason whatever as to why he could not be treated on an outpatient basis. When his East Bay Hospital psychiatrist pointed to his track record of serious suicide attempts and refused to discharge him, Greg burst into a rage and stormed out of the interview room. The next day he looked gloomy and disheveled. He was slow in both speech and movement. He confessed that he obsessed about different ways of ending his life. He favored hanging himself or asphyxiating himself in his garage. He knew he was a hopeless case—trapped forever in the painful black hole of depressive despair from which there was no escape. He was a burden to his family. They would be far better off without him.

His psychiatrist, Dr William Fischer, understood that Greg was the kind of patient who can look well enough to fool everyone. Because he could look and sound so well, he was the type of patient who usually ended up dead. That he had survived multiple suicide attempts was really a matter of luck rather than Greg's lack of suicidal intent. When he said he wanted to be dead, her very much meant it.

His treatment plan emphasized that he was a high escape risk and a moderately high suicide risk even in the hospital setting. Against his protests and threats of legal action, Greg was restricted to the locked unit of the hospital. His whereabouts and status were checked and recorded by hospital staff at fifteen-minute intervals both day and night.

His doctor and the hospital staff repeatedly told Greg that he suffered from severe depressive illness. If we could just keep him alive long enough, he would ultimately feel better and get well. Instead of giving him antidepressants, his psychiatrist opted to prescribe Zyprexa, an atypical antipsychotic drug intended to reduce his anguish and despair. Within a few days he reported that his sleep was more sound, and that his appetite had returned after months of eating in a mechanical way. Suicidal thinking was still present, but it seemed to have lost some of its force. In addition he was no longer obsessed with images of killing himself. After a week he was permitted to become a voluntary patient, and he was transferred to the unlocked unit of the hospital. Suicide precautions were changed to a less intensive level of monitoring. Despite his having made serious suicide attempts, he was no longer considered to be suicidal in the hospital. But he still needed the support of the hospital staff and treatment program, and the freedom from real and perceived responsibilities and stresses of life outside of the hospital.

He reported that he felt far less agitated. But he was still deeply depressed. Instead of anguish he now felt wiped out with no energy, no interest, and no motivation to do anything. A structured exercise and weight lifting program was added to his treatment plan. He was then started on Wellbutrin, a highly energizing antidepressant, to be taken in addition to his Zyprexa.

The focus of his psychotherapy now shifted to helping him examine how to improve his current life situation and to discourage self-recrimination about events of the past. His energy increased slowly, and he began to feel hopeful that he could do something productive for himself and his family.

Greg was ultimately discharged home. He continued to see his doctor on an outpatient basis and to take his medication as prescribed. Six months later, he got a part time job teaching in a nearby junior college.

These were the kind of patients who now almost routinely were sent to East Bay Hospital. At Walnut Creek Hospital, we had marketed ourselves as willing to treat patients who were challenging and difficult. East Bay Hospital delivered a stronger message. The message was that because of advances in the field of psychiatry, no one was any longer to be considered as untreatable. The staff at East Bay Hospital was willing and eager to treat patients who were too bizarre or too difficult for others to treat. Even if they were difficult patients with horrendous problems, they still were treatable. East Bay Hospital became known as the place that treated the undesirable. No patient was to be denied admission because of the severity of his or her mental illness. No one was considered too violent, too suicidal, or too complex to be denied treatment. Patients with complex medical and psychiatric problems were welcome.

Certain psychiatrists were more talented at treating this type of patient than others. These were therapeutic zealots who relished the challenge of what seemed to be insurmountable difficulty. Dr Alonza Johnson was one of this rare breed. He had followed us from Walnut Creek Hospital. When especially complex cases were admitted, other psychiatrists gave tribute to his skill by saying, "That is a Johnson patient. Assign that patient to Johnson's service."

"Code green–closed unit! Code green–closed unit! Code green–closed unit!" screamed the public address system. A moment later I could hear the sound of staff members running to the closed unit to help its nursing staff manage the code green situation.

A code green announcement usually meant that a violent incident had occurred or was threatened somewhere in the hospital. All hospital employees and doctors were trained to be members of the code green team. Each shift, a member of the closed unit nursing staff was assigned to be the code green team captain. When a code green was called, everyone who possibly could come would come running. The code green captain would quickly look over his pool of potential team members and make assignments. "Lois–right leg. Jim–left leg. Sandra–right arm. Georgia–left arm. I'll take the head."

The team captain would then confront the threatening patient. No one else would talk to the patient. "Jack, you are out of control. We need you to spend some time in the seclusion room until you settle down." There would only be the one statement made as clearly as possible. There would be no cajoling. There would be no argument. Often the very presence of fifteen staff members as a show of force would be sufficient. And the patient would quietly walk to the seclusion room with his arms securely grasped by two staff members.

If the patient did not cooperate with the request of the code green captain, he or she would signal, "Go!" All members of the team, almost moving as one, then quickly pinioned the violent patient to the ground. After leather straps were applied to all of his limbs, four or five staff members carried the patient into the seclusion room. He was then placed on the seclusion room bed. One limb at a time was removed from the previously applied restraints and moved to other restraints that were attached to the seclusion room bed. The patient was then given whatever medication had been ordered by the attending psychiatrist that might be appropriate for this type of emergency situation.

The patient was checked by the nursing staff at fifteen-minute intervals and the observations recorded in the patient's medical record. Once the patient had quieted sufficiently, the restraints were removed. The patient was then permitted to return to the regular closed unit area.

I always marveled at how five well-trained young women, none of who weighed more than one hundred twenty pounds, working as a team, were able to subdue almost any violent patient. Contrary to what one might imagine, injuries to staff or to patients were very few. When they did occur, they were usually minor.

I was a member of the code green teams for many years. Finally a nursing director took me aside and diplomatically explained that the nursing staff asked that I no longer participate. They reminded me that I could be of better service to the hospital in many other ways. I guessed that they thought I looked too old. Perhaps, like an aging athlete, I had slowed down and lost a step. My decreased ability to perform precisely and rapidly might be placing my fellow code green members in danger. I took their advice, but I always felt guilty when I forced myself not to respond to a "Code Green" call.

East Bay Hospital became known as the health care facility that accepted patients for treatment who had otherwise been destined for the cemetery or for the garbage heap of humanity. The staff of therapeutic zealots would provide intensive treatment for these patients over enough time to permit them to restitute to a higher level of functioning and to have some reasonable prospect of maintaining their gains. The treatment staff was always striving to help patients who at the time of discharge could be described as "the miracle of the month." Because almost all patients were considered to be candidates to become the miracle of the month, the staff excitement and intensity went into the realization of every patient's treatment plan, and a myriad of patients received an optimal level of care. It was all possible, and it was happening.

Over time the East Bay Hospital medical staff and clinical staff trained well and worked well together, intent on fixing those seen as unfixable. They believed that every patient was fixable. Their positive attitude, their energy and determination made the hospital effective. The staff exuded the aura of hope. They seemed to me the very opposite of the hopeless cynical staff who had once worked in the madhouse of Manteno. The clinical staff wanted to make what was now possible into that which was highly probable. They became a team that often produced remarkable treatment results.

While East Bay Hospital always had jealous detractors and the anti-treatment protests of civil rights activists who believed schizophrenia to be a lifestyle rather than an illness, much of the time the world loved it. A steady stream of patients from as far as one hundred fifty miles away filled the East Bay Hospital beds.

Clearly the aesthetics of the hospital were never much of a therapeutic factor. Despite our best efforts at remodeling first one wing and then another, the hospital never was beautiful. Sadly yet inevitably each newly remodeled unit received hard use from its very disturbed occupants, and signs of wear rapidly appeared. Nonetheless some patients thought East Bay Hospital the nicest place they'd ever lived in. I think they interpreted the atmosphere of kindness and hope as the physical environment of the hospital. It was really the energy, the attitude, and the training of the staff that made East Bay Hospital work.

East Bay Hospital was the fulfillment of my pledge made some forty years earlier. It was the answer to the madhouse of Manteno State Hospital. Psychiatric patients, no matter how sick or difficult they might be, could be treated in an atmosphere of kindness, respect and hope. While not everyone got well, improvement for all patients was expected and usually occurred.

In 1997 East Bay Hospital became a managed care casualty. A large number of the patients admitted to East bay Hospital were paid for by the Medicaid program. In

California, prior to 1995 hospitals that treated psychiatric patients under Medicaid directly billed the state. Hoping to save money, the state determined to pay the counties with the mental health money that had previously gone directly to all of the providers of care. The counties in turn were to contract with the non-county providers such as East Bay Hospital. It took the counties about a year to realize that if they did not send patients to non-county provider hospitals, they could keep all of the money. Dave Kears, the Director of Health Services for Alameda County, had an impossible job. He seemed to be the engine and rudder of a huge, drifting leaky barge. I liked him and respected him for his Herculean efforts. He assured me that the County decision to retain its psychiatric inpatients was, "Strictly business." Kears' line seemed straight out of *The Godfather*. I shuddered, hoping it didn't show. With false bravado I replied that Steve Heisler and I were businessmen and were used to dealing with serious business problems. But in my heart, I was terrified. This was a monster problem. In a less forthright manner other counties made the same business decision, a conspiracy of the kind that occurs every day in the business world. And within a few months the flow of patients to East Bay Hospital dropped by eighty per cent.

For a few weeks my wishes led me to think we could survive. But the spread sheets before me kept telling me something else, that the demise of the hospital was near. No matter how I manipulated the numbers and regardless of how my hopes colored my underlying assumptions, I could not figure out a formula or a strategy that would keep East Bay Hospital alive. As I viewed the imminent death of the hospital on my computer, it was like watching the speck of dust on the horizon turn into an onrushing locomotive bearing straight at me. But this time there was nothing I could do to turn it onto another track. The bottom line was that East Bay Hospital would soon be dead. Despite the quality of our clinical work, we would have to close the hospital.

Over the years my patients had taught me a great deal about feelings of failure. And I remembered all too well the feelings I had experienced from my months at Manteno State Hospital so many years earlier. At that time I had suffered from anguish and despair, although I barely recognized what was going on. Now I understood it all too clearly. Feelings of failure were a symptom, more often almost a delusional distortion of reality. They lived side by side with depression, agitation, and hopelessness. When the feeling that I was a failure hit me again, it felt like a tidal wave in which everything was turning topsy-turvy; everything collapsing on top of me. I was swimming in an ocean in which I would ultimately drown. Reality as I had known it waxed and waned. And all that was left was the raw feeling of guilt and despair.

I obsessed about what would happen to the severely ill patients who had until now found East Bay Hospital to be a haven and the embodiment of hope that they might improve, live better lives, and even get well. Would they receive intensive treatment in the County systems that had been so eager to reject them in the past? Of course not! They would end up in the revolving door system, receiving Band-Aid care only to quickly regress and reappear a short time later for another round. Some would join the statistic of successful suicides. Others would get lost on the streets and in flop houses living a subhuman psychotic existence.

I hurt for them. By day I went about my business with a heavy heart barely contained in my tightened chest. My appetite disappeared, and my sleep was miserable. At night and on weekends I curled up in a ball to try to reduce the pain I felt throughout my body. I knew very well it was all tension and that lying in bed only made things worse. It was the worst thing that I could do. For decades I had been pushing depressed patients to get out of bed. The apparent comfort of the bed was a trap that only amplified feelings of depression and thoughts of failure. My own pain underscored how right I had been during all of my years as a clinician.

My wife, Melanie, literally dragged me out of bed and took me for long walks—which helped. She listened to my obsessive thoughts about the problems of the hospital and the patients who would no longer be treated there. She firmly told me I wasn't a failure, and she encouraged me in a thousand ways. One of my sons, John, gave me a stuffed monkey which when squeezed said things like "You're brilliant!" "You're wonderful!" "Good job!" "Great idea!" While laughing at myself, I squeezed it a lot.

Once I accepted the inevitable fate of the hospital, I felt much less pain than when I had been thrashing about seeking a solution that wasn't there. The pain was replaced by a dull sense of resignation. I turned my attention to writing a plan for closing the hospital. The plan included hundreds of steps of what had to be done and when it had to be done. How different from opening a hospital. Opening the hospital had been fun. There had been confusion, problems galore, excitement and irritability along with enthusiasm and hope. The future brought a bright glow and extended indefinitely forward. In stark contrast closing the hospital was deliberate, carefully scripted and finite, all in an atmosphere of depression, resentment and hopelessness.

After the hospital closed down, Steve Heisler and I developed a better perspective on what had happened. East Bay Hospital had been a great adventure. Despite our own business skill deficiencies, it had proven possible to provide psychiatric care for even the most seriously ill psychiatric patients. The example of East Bay Hospital proved that it was now possible for the vast majority to feel better and function better.

Steve looked back and recalled the misery of trying to operate an under-funded hospital. He also recalled East Bay Hospital as the most high-powered intensive care unit for psychiatry in all of Northern California. He was sad that the hospital closed, yet relieved at his new-found freedom from stress.

I too remember my sleepless nights, the physical pain of total body tension, the sense of dread, our days of depression and the innumerable political and fiscal challenges. But I also think about how proud I was to say that I had been one of the founders of East Bay Hospital and to describe our challenging clinical work in saving very ill patients from the nightmare of mental illness.

Steve and I continued as partners in psychiatric office practice. Apart from seeing patients at our offices, we did consulting work for hospital companies in the United States and England. Occasionally we talked about battles won and defeats endured in the hospital business. We recalled the incredibly sick patients who were treated at East Bay Hospital and our staff's success in helping them. More often we marveled at the field of psychiatry as it had been transformed, at what could be done today that not too long ago was unclear or impossible. We still became excited when we saw troubled people feel better, function better and become able to make better choices to improve their lives. And as clinicians we were pleased to take part in the day to day treatment of our patients, a painstaking and at times frustrating process through which the great puzzles in psychiatric treatment come closer to solution.

XVIII. GOOD-BYE MADHOUSE

One morning I was searching the internet, look-ing for information about the fate of Manteno State Hospital and other megalithic state mental hospitals like Manteno. An advertisement for a rock concert gave me a sudden jolt. I hadn't been expecting it at all. It read something like, "John Stone and the Pluggers at Brownstone Psychiatric Hospital." The advertisement was followed by a dozen pictures taken at the concert showing animated musicians and an entranced audi-ence, all with the main building of Brownstone Hospital, looking like an eerie Gothic castle, forming a surreal and awesome background.

Brownstone, a crumbling, decomposing, yet still handsome structure, was now shuttered and in total disrepair. It was one of those many state hospitals like Manteno that just a half century ago had each ware-housed thousands of mentally ill patients.

It was so strange to see the hospital looking like this. The hospital as a living organism wasn't really there. The memories of the horrors that patients endured (and sometimes couldn't endure) were barely there, having morphed into a kind of gruesome stage set, a creepy ghoulish joke, a gigantic Halloween party setting that makes us laugh and smile at death and torture rather than feel dread, terror, and sorrow.

The happy rock concert at Brownstone seemed so much at odds with the reality of patient neglect and abuse that at first I was sickened and offended at what I was seeing. It was like having a carnival at the site of a World War II concentration camp.

After a few minutes of agonizing I began to see the whole rock concert scene from a very different perspective. At least for me the rock concert became a kind of celebration, a party celebrating that the hospital was closed, that the madhouse with all its ugliness and pathos was no more.

But one has to be careful not to get carried away. In our wishful thinking it is all too easy to pretend to ourselves that mental illness is no longer with us, that it doesn't really exist anymore.

The closure of the megalithic state psychiatric hospitals does not mean that those afflicted by psychotic illness have magically disappeared. Psychiatric hospitals are still very necessary, although now the facilities are reasonably pleasant, more often like mid-level motels. And the lengths of stay for the vast majority of patients are relatively brief and for the most part happily crowned with a positive outcome after days or weeks of intensive treatment. A few high security facilities still exist to house those whose illnesses have been refractory to even the best of the treatments we have today.

But what about the rest of those patients with serious mental illness who refuse treatment or for whom treatment is unavailable? They have been dumped onto the city streets to become a small army of panhandlers who live a subhuman existence in doorways, cardboard boxes, and flophouses. While no longer incarcerated, they are still imprisoned in the bizarre world of chronic mental illness. For now, except for their more egregious lapses into peculiar or threatening behavior, the presence of the mentally ill on the city streets seems all too well tolerated. Society no longer seems to need (or is unable) to sweep these sufferers from chronic mental illness off the streets and into treatment facilities where they have a chance to get well. Instead our apparent tolerance, a product of a societal exhaustion of funds and resources, has fostered a serious neglect that requires major change. Even with all of our advances in treatment, the problem has not gone away.

XIX. COMING SOON TO YOUR LOCAL SHRINK

It is thrilling that the madhouse is gone. It is even more exciting that the science in psychiatry has given us pharmacological tools to help manage and even cure many mental conditions. The vast majority of those with mental illness are now able to lead almost symptom free, productive and happy lives. And it is satisfying that after years of political struggle, new parity legislation on a national level is mandating that insurance carriers provide better coverage for any of us who seek or require psychiatric care.

So what is next? What is new on the mental health horizon?

Like the erosion of a river bed, the further evolution of psychiatry is an almost invisible process, too gradual for us to see day by day. If we pause to think about it, we may see some changes from year to year—less frequent, though, through the use of the new miraculous drugs than we might imagine.

The changes in the field of psychiatry rarely come as a result of 'definitive' university studies or drug company-financed research projects. Most of the time the changes come about through psychiatrists' painstaking efforts to learn to use psychiatric drugs that have been newly introduced or those that are already available. Once a new drug is developed, prompted by a sense of therapeutic zeal, we begin the process of using it occasionally in our day to day clinical work whenever it seems appropriate—especially when it seems that for a given patient other more established drugs are not working well. From our patients' experience and from our colleagues' anecdotal accounts exchanged during lunch time or corridor conversations, we then learn bits of valuable clinical information. It often turns out that the most effective uses of new or even older drugs is not even close to those descriptions and instructions provided when the drugs first were FDA approved and brought to the marketplace. For example, Abilify, originally prescribed for psychotic illness, turned out not to live up to expectations. But with our patients' help we discovered that it is an excellent drug when used as an andjunct to antidepressant medications. To our professional satisfaction and our patients' happy surprise, we come to understand that many drugs may be most useful when given in different dosages or in combinations with other medications. And sometimes old drugs are revisited and found to be more effective than our previous understanding would have indicated.

Scientific studies that corroborate what clinicians have come to understand from their day to day experience may not be published till years later. The announcement of a new FDA approved use of a drug often causes almost a yawn by the myriads of practicing psychiatrists who had come to know the "new indication" years earlier in their own day to day clinical work.

Based on what is going on now, let me make some predictions about what will become commonplace in clinical practice over the next decade.

1.   Lower Suicide Rates

Most suicide attempts are preceded by periods of anguish and despair. Patients describe these feelings as a kind of pain so severe that escape from life appears to be the only avenue for relief. They feel trapped in a nightmare from which they cannot wake up. Many describe this state of torment as feeling trapped in an all encompassing painful black hole with no prospect of relief. To them living is truly Hell, and death seems the only possible escape from torture.

The great news is that anguish and despair can now be controlled, decreased and even eliminated, with at least some degree of relief most often within a day or two! When anguish and despair disappear, the drive to commit suicide fades rapidly. A number of members of a class of somewhat unrelated psychiatric medications, known as atypical antipsychotic drugs, can provide such wonderful relief that what were once almost obsessive thoughts of suicide become less intense, less frequent, and then just disappear. Patients often comment later how they had seemed to be stuck in an abysmal world of negative thinking and painful feelings with no prospect of escape, and that medication in an almost magical way changed their whole outlook almost over night.

These medications, such as Risperdal, Zyprexa, Geodon, Invega, Fanapt or Seroquel, were all initially developed to treat schizophrenia. While not antidepressant drugs, their role in escape from the black hole nightmare brings with it an incredible sense of relief. And the drive to end one's life rapidly becomes yesterday's soon to be forgotten bad dream.

2.   Safer and More Effective Use of Antidepressant Drugs.

Many antidepressant drugs often do not seem to improve anguish and despair. Admittedly some antidepressant drugs, such as Prozac and Wellbutrin, may at times actually worsen a sense of psychological pain. And with that increased inner torment comes suicidal thinking, even suicide attempts. These well publicized charges often frighten patients not to seek medical help for severe depression, or parents to refuse to have their children of any age take the antidepressants their doctors may have prescribed.

Our improved understanding both of depression and of antidepressant drugs helps us to employ antidepressant medications far more safely and much more effectively than before.

We psychiatrists have always known that depressions are not all the same. But in the past we did not appreciate that a simple classification might have extremely important consequences in determining an optimal choice of effective medications. Those depressions characterized by lack of energy, excess sleep, and little motivation can be termed 'apathetic' depressions. Those that feature sleeplessness, agitation, irritability, anguish and despair along with suicidal ideation can be called 'agitated' depressions. These are very different conditions and respond differently to different antidepressant medications.

We can also distinguish one antidepressant from another by how energizing they may be. Some are very sedating, while others may be very energizing. Apathetic depressions respond well to energizing antidepressants. These very same energizing antidepressants may make agitated depressions worse—with increased suicidal ideation. Patients with agitated depression respond much more favorably to calming or sedating antidepressants, especially when they are used along with atypical antipsychotic mood stabilizers (as described earlier). Just this simple classification of depressed patients into one of several types enables us clinicians to more effectively and safely choose the most helpful antidepressants for our patients.

3.   A New But Old Family of Antidepressants Makes a Comeback

An old family of powerful antidepressant drugs, known as the MAOI (mono amine oxidase inhibitors) class for decades had been vilified and almost forgotten—except as a warning sign on most drug information labels. A whole generation of psychiatrists has had no training and little if any experience in their use. Most doctors have even forgotten what the problem with MAOI drugs had been in the first place.

The danger with MAOI drugs can be a sudden increase in blood pressure at times leading to a stroke, but only when they are used along with certain foods or other medications. What has been less clear is that there are several types of MAOI drugs, one group of which is harmless. For the other group, Marplan, Nardil and Parnate, the forbidden foods list is very short and easily followed. But the dietary restrictions are far less rigid than once envisioned.

This family of drugs may be helpful when many other antidepressants have been tried and have failed. A comeback in the use of both groups of MAOI antidepressants has already begun. A not so new and very safe MAOI, selegeline, some years ago became available as a skin patch, Emsam. No more effective and no more safe than the oral form, its availability reminds us that the tablet form has been around for many years. Both seem harmless, even without adherence to the moderately restrictive diet mandated when other MAOI drugs are prescribed.

Patients find that there is little problem with safe usage of the drugs and often look back and wonder what all the fuss had been about. More often they are pleased with their effectiveness and relative freedom from the weight gain and sexual dysfunction side effects commonly seen as side effects of the more popular antidepressant drugs.

4. Improving Memory

Those medications already available for ameliorating the intellective deficit of Alzheimer's Disease turn out to help memory defects related to other problems as well. Many antidepressant drugs, used alone or in combination with other medications, often produce some degree of recent memory defect, problems with concentration, or difficulty in coming up with the right word or name. Medications such as Exelon, Aricept, and Namenda can produce significant relief in a very short time. Tenex, developed to treat high blood pressure, is now used to treat attention deficit disorder in children and adults. It, too, is helpful for improving concentration and memory problems that result from any number of causes.

It is a tantalizing dream that we all can become smarter if we take medication that helps improve intellective functioning. But that day may not be that far away.

5. Some Alcoholics Might Become Social Drinkers

Ideally alcoholics should stop drinking completely and use a 12-step program to help maintain sobriety. But in real life most of them won't even consider the idea. They deny that they have an alcohol problem that they cannot control. One unique medication, Campral, helps reduce the craving for alcohol to a significant degree. Once they start taking Campral on a daily basis, some alcoholics will actually stop drinking. Others can control the amount they drink, albeit with some degree of conscious struggle. When they take Campral every day, often to their surprise they encounter a sense that "a few is enough." And their substantially reduced total intake may be sufficient to change the course of their lives. Without the Campral many of these alcoholics were otherwise destined to have their lives implode with loss of jobs and families.

6.   Weight Loss Without Danger

All dieters know that stimulants help to reduce appetite for a short time. But within days or weeks their appetites are screaming again. Increased dosages of stimulants bring about unpleasant and even dangerous side effects such as elevated blood pressure, insomnia, irritability, agitation and paranoid thinking.

But not all appetite reducing drugs are stimulants. A side effect of one non-stimulant medication, Topomax, originally developed to treat seizure disorders, turns out to enable moderate appetite reduction and weight loss. Taken according to a particular dosing schedule, Topomax provides effective appetite reduction for many dieters. Wellbutrin, an energizing antidepressant, may also reduce appetite when used in therapeutic dosages.

All these pharmacologic tools and more are actually with us. Over the next decade their usage will become more widespread. And just around the corner are new antidepressants with less impact on appetite and a lower incidence of sexual dysfunction. New antipsychotic medications will have fewer side effects and will be more energizing. Obsessive compulsive disorders will respond to new combinations of drugs that will provide far better symptom control. And even Alzheimer's Disease will be more effectively arrested.

Wow! I can't wait!